THE GIRLFRIENDS' GUIDE TO EMPTY NESTING

THE GIRLFRIENDS' GUIDE TO EMPTY NESTING

Allie Hill

Finn-Phyllis
Press

Copyright © 2024 by Allie Hill

All rights reserved. No part of this publication may be reproduced, in whole or in part, in any form or by any means, electronic or mechanical, including photocopying, recording, or by any information gathering storage and retrieval system now known or hereafter invented, without written permission from the publisher.

Published by Finn-Phyllis Press

www.FinnPhyllisPress.com

ISBN 979-8-9873612-8-3 (paperback)
ISBN 979-8-9873612-7-6 (eBook)

First Edition

The author of this book is not a physician or a licensed therapist. She does not prescribe the use of any technique as a form of treatment for physical, emotional, or medical problems without the advice of a physician, directly or indirectly. The intent of the author is only to offer information of a general nature to help you in your quest for emotional, physical, and spiritual well-being. The author and publisher assume no liability for damages caused as a result of using the ideas or suggestions in this book. Some names have been changed for privacy purposes.

To Jim and Isabella, Bosley and Bear. I love you!

CONTENTS

Introducion i

01: Where's the Bleeping Manual? 1

02: Saying Goodbye
(Without Having a Breakdown) 7

03: Why So Far Away? 19

04: Step One: Be Good to Yourself 27

05: The Truth About Who You Are
(and Who You'll Become) 41

06: So…Now What?! 51

07: Is It Time to Get a Cat? 61

08: All the Time in the World
(and Not in a Good Way) 67

09: Creating Connection (Outside Social Media) 73

10: Where Do I Hang My Mom Hat
(and What Do I Wear Instead)? 79

11: Communicating With Adult(ish) Kids 95

12: Enter Menopause: Hormone Hell
(and Other Rude Double-Whammies) 105

13: Who Am I Married To? 111

14: Too Much of a Good Thing(?) 125

15: Where are Rachel, Monica, and Phoebe
When I Need Them? 137

16: I've Got 99 Problems
      (and You're Still 85 of Them) 147

17: Yay, You're Home!
      (How Long Did You Say You're Staying?) 151

18: All the Single Ladies: Put Your Hands Up! 161

19: So…Now What (Again)? 169

ACKNOWLEDGMENTS 171

ABOUT THE AUTHOR 175

INTRODUCTION

"If you are brave enough to say goodbye, life will reward you with a new hello."
—*Paulo Coelho*

First of all, I'm so glad you're here.

If you're at all like I was after our daughter, Izzy (our only child), left for college, you're experiencing a whole lot of feelings: pride, sadness, excitement, uncertainty, worry, possibly even anxiety or depression.

Whether you dropped off a kid at college in the last few days, or all of your children have been out of the house for weeks (or years), the tsunami of emotions swirling in your body is a result of having wholly devoted yourself to the most honorable and underappreciated career path in the world: motherhood—and not being at all sure what comes after that.

I want you to know that all these feelings are normal.

You picked up this book because you're ready to stop feeling empty, purposeless, or uncertain about the future. You're ready for hope, and you're open to possibilities. I don't have a crystal ball, so I cannot tell you precisely what your future holds, but I know it can be just as unique, fulfilling, and joy-filled as it was when you had your children under your roof 24/7, if not more so! But if you're feeling a bit skeptical about what's next, I understand.

It's important to acknowledge that your child, or children, embarking on their own independent adventure indicates that you've done your job as a parent, and that's worth celebrating! I mean, it's not like you didn't do anything for the last twenty years. Even if you don't have millions of dollars in the bank, a building named after you, or something otherwise tangible to show for all your years of work, you raised human beings. You didn't get to the point where you said, "Keep the dorm room (or apartment) clean" and "Make good choices, please, for the love of God" by accident. Think of all the hundreds of hours you poured into these tiny beings until they were ready to brave the world by themselves.

That, my friend, is a miracle.

Not only did you spend the last eighteen to twenty-plus years taking care of every minute detail of these young beings' lives, but you also had a full nine months to prepare for their arrival. Why is it that, just when they are on the cusp of adulthood, a complex phase of the parent/child relationship, there's so little information and guidance available on how to do this?

You've spent the last twenty years caring for everyone and everything around you. Your sole focus has been the health and well-being of your family. For the first time in decades, you are not obliged to be singularly focused. Even though you will always have an "ear to the ground" in anticipating your adult child's needs, you are being asked to let go and allow them to be an adult, and even further, to find your passion and fulfillment outside the family.

When I dropped our daughter off at college six years ago, I couldn't find a single book on navigating the empty-nest journey. To say that I struggled would be an immense understatement. In truth, my struggle began when my daughter was a junior in high school, and the prospect of her going off to college, although two years away, was already daunting. Having an only child and putting "all of my eggs in one basket" created a laser-focus devotion to her and all that raising her entailed.

I remember spring break of her junior year of high school. I was driving Izzy and her friend Skye to dinner, and "Leaving on a Jet Plane" by John Denver came on the radio. Out of nowhere, I burst into tears. My daughter looked at me, horrified, and asked, "What's the matter?" I told her the song reminded me that she and her friend would be leaving for college in two years, and it was more than I could bear. As dramatic as it may sound, there were numerous times over the course of those two years when a particular song or activity nearly took my breath away as we inched closer and closer to D-Day (Departure Day).

Her senior year, when she and her friends were beginning to get a whiff of freedom and independence, felt like the longest, saddest goodbye to me. Everything represented "the last": the last Homecoming, the last bonfire, the last pep rally, the last Thanksgiving Day parade, the last Christmas break, the last spring break, the last prom.

Each of these "lasts" felt like a ten-pound brick stacked on my heart. And, as my heart became heavier, my daughter's heart only seemed to become lighter with each passing month, the thought of freedom and independence like a hot air balloon whisking her away from our home (a home she indicated on numerous occasions felt increasingly like a prison).

I made hundreds of mistakes in those first eighteen years raising my daughter, but surely, I made ninety-two percent of them during her junior and senior years. I realize now that the more tightly I gripped and tried to assert my control, the more she rebelled and tried to declare her independence. In retrospect, some of my mistakes were funny, like when I offered to host her high school graduation party. I imagined having it at the neighborhood barn where the kids grew up swimming and riding horses. It would be a super casual, no-muss-no-fuss situation. That is, until my daughter's friend posted the invitation on Facebook, and what started as twenty to thirty kids and parents quickly turned into 200, then 400, kids from all over the city. I asked my husband what I should do, and he suggested

I contact our local police department to hire some off-duty police officers to help, as my primary concern was kids drinking and driving.

I called the local police station, and Officer Stu took my call. I explained my predicament, and he told me that the station no longer offered off-duty police officers, as there seemed to be a conflict of interest between the parents' wishes and the actual law. When I asked him to clarify, he said, "They want us around, but if their kids drink, they want us to turn a blind eye. It doesn't make any sense."

I asked what he would do if he were in my position. "Cancel it!" he said without hesitation. And so I did. This decision did not make me immensely popular with my daughter, her friends, or her friends' parents, who were counting on me to host the party and take on all the responsibility. Instead, I co-hosted a simple graduation party at a nearby park. Let it be said that, by this point, the kids had been celebrating their pending graduation at other friends' parties for two weeks already, so by the time our party rolled around, two of them had mono, and most of the rest were exhausted.

I have learned so much in the six years since my daughter's first year of college. I have been coaching soon-to-be and newly empty-nest moms for over three years, and I have learned that although each of our journeys is unique, we all face the same uncertain future and are looking for the same answers to "Okay, now what?!" The book you're reading is the one I wish I had found when I began my empty-nest journey. I write it as both a tribute to my own journey and a gift to you, my beloved reader.

I hope this book serves as a guide, a roadmap for finding out what is important to you now, and where you want to spend your time and attention. I set out to write a book that is both useful and lighthearted. I want you to feel seen and heard in the stories you read and discover practical strategies and tools to help you design the next chapter of your amazing life. I also hope it compels you to reconnect with yourself and remember who you are as well as who you've always wanted to be. I am cheering you on, and I hope you will use the tools and strategies to connect to and align with your values and purpose.

By opening this book, you are taking the first step in imagining your new path forward. You are actively creating an extraordinary life, one in which you can feel just as fulfilled as you did as a full-time parent.

To be clear, this book is not intended to be the definitive guide for empty nesters. Rather, think of it exactly as the title describes: "The Girlfriends' Guide to Empty-Nesting"—a compendium of things that worked (and didn't), as well as some practical tips, tools, and suggestions that have helped my friends, clients, and myself.

We will talk through where you are now on your empty-nest journey and, even more importantly, where you want to go (and how to get there). I'll be sure to let you in on some solid strategies for managing your understandable feelings of sadness, uncertainty, and overwhelm. I promise, the road before you is wide open, and the possibilities are endless.

TOP 6 TIPS AS YOU PREPARE FOR THE EMPTY NEST

Expand your Hobbies & Interests

One of the most important things to remember as you prepare for the empty nest is the importance of fostering interests and passions beyond parenting. Whether it's basket weaving, a fascination with reptiles, or the art of making sourdough bread, having diverse hobbies will enrich your life and ensure a fulfilling existence outside of raising your children.

Be Open to Uncomfortable Conversations

During your child's junior and senior years of high school, conversations often revolve around life post-high school. It's an incredibly high-pressure time for our kids, and focusing solely on what they're going to do after graduation only intensifies that pressure. Make an effort to engage in a wide variety of conversation topics and consider designating a specific time, say Sundays at 5PM, when you officially check in with them about their future. This will help ensure deeper safety and connection between you and your kids.

Value Your Child's Unique Journey

While higher education is often considered a milestone, it's crucial to refrain from imposing the idea of attending university on your child if they have no interest. Each individual has unique talents and passions, and it is vital to support their chosen path, whether it involves pursuing a trade, entrepreneurship, or any other avenue that aligns with their aspirations.

Celebrate Achievements Mindfully

Should your child receive a college acceptance, it's natural to be overjoyed and relieved. However, it's essential to remember that not all achievements are comparable. Avoid the temptation to publicly announce their college acceptance in a manner that may inadvertently upset them or overshadow or undermine the achievements of others. (Please refer to chapter 2 for the details on how I included United Airlines in my announcement of Izzy's college acceptance, much to her dismay.)

Take Your Time When Redoing Kids' Rooms

Whether your child is heading off to college or permanently moving out of the home, it's a time of big transition for them, and there are a few adjustments that they perhaps aren't ready to (and don't have to) make just yet. Coming home to discover that their room has been turned into a yoga studio or an overflow for your closet can be jarring. If possible, keep their room as it is for their first year away. It's comforting for kids when home feels predictable, safe, and certain. Also, begin conversations with your adult children about your plans for future room renovations. This gives them some time to warm up to the idea. Of course, it's always your prerogative to do what you want with your home, but allowing a grace period where they have at least one change-free environment can go a long way.

Resist the Urge to Compare

It is almost impossible not to compare how your child is doing with how your friends' kids are reportedly doing. Comparing situations is human nature, but it can be detrimental to both your child's well-being and your own. Each individual has a unique journey, and comparing their choices or achievements to those of others only diminishes the joy and happiness that should accompany their personal growth. Embrace the diversity of experiences and celebrate each individual's path.

The more you can allow your child to have their own journey and not fret if it doesn't look like that of your neighbor's kid, the better. The truth is, even the kid who got into Yale (on a full ride) and was the first freshman to start on the rowing team could still be struggling with making friends, managing anxiety, or dealing with the pressure to make his parents proud. To the best of your ability, stay in your own lane, and know that in most cases, everything is working out just as it should.

CHAPTER 1

Where's the Bleeping Manual?

"I think the hardest thing for a mother is to make it possible for a child to be independent and at the same time let the child know how much you love her, how much you want to take care of her, and yet how truly essential it is for her to fly on her own."
—*Madeleine Albright*

One of the first things moms wonder when their kids leave home (for whatever reason) is "How do I do life after this?"

When I began my empty-nest journey, I felt like a shell of my former self, completely empty inside, as though my identity had evaporated overnight. In many ways, it had. After all, women with three or four kids (or even two) aren't ushered so violently into the empty-nest journey. They get to ease into it. But in my case, one day I was a full-time mom, and the next day I wasn't. I realized very quickly (and a bit too late) that I'd never taken the time to think about Act Two. It quickly became apparent that I would need a lot of help "filling my well" in order to establish a new sense of purpose and fulfillment.

I recognized that many of my close friends and family members expected me to have figured out how to navigate this new chapter and know what the next part of my life looked like. Further, those who were also preparing to embark upon the empty-nest journey seemed to know exactly what *they* were doing next, and they were surprised when I expressed that I didn't. In fact, I had a slew of well-meaning friends who frequently looked at me with concerned expressions, asking, "No, but really, what *are* you going to do when Izzy goes off to college?" Surprisingly, I realized that even *I* expected I'd somehow "just know" what the next chapter would look like. But the time had come. And I didn't.

I thought about getting an apartment next to Izzy's school, but she didn't believe that was nearly as good of an idea as I did (shocker!). I thought about going back to school myself, writing a book, learning Latin, or taking up knitting. What I knew for sure was that I didn't *only* want to join a tennis, golf, or book club, and I *did* want to help, inspire, and empower other women. But I had no idea how to make that my new reality.

(More about figuring out what you *do* want in chapter 3).

Before long, it became necessary to open myself up to the possibility that I could indeed create an exciting second half of my life. Acknowledging that possibility was my first step, and soon after, I could feel a subtle shift in my energy and my attitude towards my future. For the first time in almost twenty years, I realized that my time was once again my own. The thought of life being a blank canvas was both exciting and scary, but my renewed perspective allowed me to wake up excited to see what each day would bring. I was ever so slowly becoming a person who could at least entertain the idea that this next chapter might hold some joy and happiness, and I was committed to staying open to all the possibilities that lay ahead.

Many people wonder, "How do I pivot so abruptly? How do I create Act Two out of thin air?" It's important to point out that you can use the same skills and determination that got you through the eighteen-plus years of raising your child(ren) to create the next chapter of your life.

Think about how you used to make a schedule or fill a calendar with activities so you'd know who was doing what on each day and at what time, what equipment they'd need, when they'd be picked up, and when you'd need to have food ready for them when they got home. We are used to juggling many balls and being problem-solvers and cheerleaders, and truthfully, very few problems have ever arisen that we couldn't find a solution to.

It's time to invest the same clarity, determination, ability to prioritize and execute, and follow-through you've devoted to your family, friends, and community into yourself. That's how you'll find out who you are now, at this moment in your life, and nurture that. That typically feels foreign, and as a result, it makes many of us quite uncomfortable. After all, we're used to doing for others and putting ourselves last.

I know it's been a long time since you focused on your likes, desires, dreams, and hobbies. You're understandably out of practice.

I'll let you in on a little secret: The more you can tend to your own garden, so to speak, the greater joy and relief your life partner and children will feel. What they want most is for you to be happy, fulfilled, and content, not sitting in bed all day with scrapbooks from your kids' first years and four boxes of Kleenex. I say this as someone who spent the first few weeks at home after dropping Izzy off wandering aimlessly from room to room, not sure what I was looking for but knowing I felt lost and unmoored.

"But how do I do that?" you're no doubt asking. For goodness' sake, it's easier to find 176 YouTube videos on how to fix your clogged garbage disposal than it is to find information on how to successfully transition into life as an empty nester. I easily found at least twenty books on what to expect before, during, and after I was expecting, but a straightforward book on empty-nesting that wasn't largely Bible-based or steeped in cognitive-based-therapy jargon? That was hard to come by.

When it comes to why there aren't more books, support options, and discussions about this tricky transition in life, I believe it's because we, as moms, are used to handling all our problems ourselves—often internally. Culturally, there seems to be a bit of shame associated with needing some help and guidance. I find this to be true in general, but especially when kids leave the home.

Collectively, we spend years preparing our kids for college but don't spend the same time and attention preparing the parents! Whoever invented the SAT and ACT should also have created the ENSC (the Empty-Nest Survival Course). I would have taken it at least twice! Ours isn't the first generation of mothers to feel a tremendous sense of loss in the areas of identity and purpose when our kids leave home. Many celebrities, including Brooke Shields and Kelly Ripa, have proclaimed to the world how painful this experience was for them, normalizing the often-challenging process of letting our kids go.

It's a conundrum: You spend decades raising humans, hoping and praying you've prepared them to go off into the world. But when they do, you swiftly realize that in the process of teaching them how to be adults, you forgot about *you*! Where is *your* guidance counselor? Who is helping you figure out *your* next steps, how you want to spend your time, and what life looks like post-twenty-four-hour-a-day mommying?

Let's get started with what's often the most challenging part: saying goodbye.

CHAPTER 2

Saying Goodbye (Without Having a Breakdown)

"Give the ones you love wings to fly, roots to come back, reasons to stay."
—*Dalai Lama*

Letting go is an interesting—and sometimes lightning-rod—topic.

Some of my highest engagement on social media comes from my posts on letting go. Some women feel like "letting go" of their kids is impossible because it seems to go against their innate motherly instincts. I completely understand this feeling because, remember, I'm the girl who looked into moving across state lines to be nearer to my daughter.

It makes sense that it's hard to let go. After so much time devoted to these lovely beings, you're now supposed to just drop the reins? The real question is, how do we go from controlling every aspect of our children's lives to letting go completely? How do we allow them not only to make their own decisions but also watch as they make mistakes without immediately jumping in to try to fix everything?

Let's face it. As mothers, we micromanage, for the most part, our kids' lives from birth through the mid-teenage years. So whether we choose to hit the eject button the second they graduate or opt for a slower weaning process, we all realize at some point that we were never really in control in the first place. Therefore, the sooner we empower our children to take care of themselves, the better off they (and we) will be.

I am going to recuse myself from the start by admitting that I had lots of trouble letting go of control (if you haven't already figured that out!). I may or may not have asked my daughter's doctor if we could microchip her before her departure.

Izzy loves to tell a story about me collecting her friends' cell phones when she had sleepovers. I think the underlying reason she loves telling this story is that it reminds her of the instances when she felt she had the opportunity to "be the adult." Apparently, my requests for everyone's phones were tolerable when she was in middle school, but they became embarrassing and bordered on harassment once they were in high school.

As we neared the time when she would be leaving

for college, Izzy looked at me one day before her friends arrived for the night and said, "Mom, I'm almost eighteen years old, and I'm going off to college, where I will have literally no rules and no one telling me what to do. How about I practice this summer while I'm still at home?"

Mic drop!

I hadn't noticed that I was holding on so tightly to my nearly adult daughter, whom I still thought of as being nine years old. Cell phone management was but one of many examples of the ways I was trying to control her (all for her own well-being, of course!).

I still booked all of her doctor and dentist appointments, automobile checkups, and anything else that involved any level of planning, cost, or impact to my schedule.

The other day, I spoke to a friend who told me she was having this very dilemma. Her nineteen-year-old son was having pain in his left testicle. Because he was clearly in pain, she wanted to resolve the situation as quickly as possible. "He's uncomfortable making the appointment and talking about his testicle," she told me, "but his dad believes he's old enough to make his own doctor appointments."

Izzy is now twenty-four years old, and it's safe to say that she makes ninety percent of her doctor appointments. One reason this particular transition was a bit easier was that she began being more in charge of this area of her life when she was home from college for part of 2020 during the pandemic. She needed to see a dentist, and I suggested that since she knew her schedule best, she should make her appointment. Being in charge of such matters has worked pretty well for the last few years, however she doesn't live in the same state as we do, where her previous doctors are, and sometimes things fall through the cracks. I sometimes still feel like a dorm mom, constantly checking in to see if she has followed up on making necessary appointments.

On the other hand, Izzy had a good friend named Annie who seemed to come out of the womb as a young adult. She was balancing her checkbook and keeping a strict budget in middle school. She was even proactively reminding her parents of the need to schedule her bi-annual dentist appointment. So impressed with her adulting skills at such an early age, I asked her mother to share how she got her daughter to take on so many mature responsibilities when I couldn't get mine to do so much as make her bed, feed the dog, or do her laundry.

"I think Annie likes feeling responsible and knowing she can take care of herself," her mother shared. "She has always been an old soul. I'm not sure I did anything particularly special, but I showed her how, and she was internally motivated to take on these responsibilities."

For kids who aren't as proactive about taking responsibility for these tasks (and for moms who are maintaining these responsibilities to hold on to the last vestiges of their maternal duties), letting go of trying to control everything is a daunting task, and the struggle to let go might even show up in unexpected places.

It was a Thursday afternoon in mid-March 2017 when our phones started pinging. Izzy and I were walking through the shoe department at Nordstrom, perusing sandals for an upcoming trip to California.

Izzy quickly checked her phone and announced the first message out loud: "Skye got into CU!" And then the second: "Annie got into CU and University of Arizona!" And then the third: "Kyla got into Colorado University and Colorado State!" The list kept going.

She plopped down on a bench to check her email—no word on her admissions status. Of the fourteen colleges and universities throughout the country she'd applied to, she hadn't heard back from a single one.

I told her to pocket her phone, and we headed to another store. "Nothing a little retail therapy can't help," I thought.

But the niggling thought persisted in the back of my mind. *What if she doesn't get into a single college?* It had never dawned on me that she might *not* attend college in the fall.

Izzy had diligently prepared for her ACTs and SATs. She had met with her college counselor, who suggested she apply to a combination of easy, medium, and "reach" schools. I thought we'd checked all the boxes. But there we were, waiting in limbo.

I tried to channel my nervous energy into optimism. "No worries, honey," I said, attempting to be comforting. "You will get into the college you're supposed to get into. It will all work out in the end."

Months earlier, we had planned to visit the L.A. area with my friend Kim and her daughter Skye to check out Southern California schools the girls were interested in. I was happy for the upcoming distraction.

When we got on the plane, Kim and I sat toward the front, and the girls were a few rows behind us. We happily chatted about our plan for the next few days, and how we would balance school visits with beach time and fun.

When we touched down in L.A., I grabbed my phone to text the girls our next steps, and that's when I saw Izzy's text:

OMG! Mom! I got into U of A!

I actually screamed out loud. And then I started scream-crying, hard enough that I couldn't even tell Kim what was happening. I just kept shaking my phone at her as I cried tears of joy. And relief! My dramatic reaction did not go unnoticed. A concerned flight attendant quickly made a beeline to ensure I was okay.

"Yes," I stammered between sobs. "I just found out my daughter got in to college!"

She looked relieved (though perhaps a bit perplexed), smiled at me, and said, "That's terrific! I'm so glad; you had me worried there for a second!"

I'd stopped crying and was basking in complete

euphoria, which is the only reason I can imagine I had the thought to ask, "Do you think you could make an announcement? I'd like to give my daughter a big congratulations. It will be such a fun surprise!"

At this point, my enthusiasm was contagious, and the flight attendant nodded her head. Who doesn't want to be the bearer of good news?

"Welcome to L.A. You may retrieve your baggage on carousel 8. Please look around to ensure you have all your belongings before departing the plane. We have a special announcement to make. Let's all give a big round of applause to…" She covered the microphone.

"Isabella Hill!" I shouted.

"Isabella Hill," she continued. "She just found out she was accepted to the University of…" She again covered the mic.

"Arizona!" I yelled, like it was Harvard!

"Ok then…Arizona! Congratulations!" she concluded.

I was nearly apoplectic, whistling, clapping, and smiling from ear to ear. My flight mates, on the other hand, were less enthused. Some gave a rather pathetic slow clap and hurried off the plane, giving me the side-eye as they departed.

I was so overjoyed and, truthfully, relieved, that I wanted to share my joy with the entire airplane. I wanted my daughter to know how proud I was of her accomplishment and how excited I was for her news.

Kim looked at me with mixed emotions. She was mostly laughing, and I could tell that she applauded my enthusiasm, but there was something more. She was also shaking her head, a subtle nod to her prediction that my daughter would be less than happy about my choice to celebrate in this way.

Kim and I disembarked first and waited for the girls. I thought that perhaps if I committed to the emotion of joy, maybe it would be contagious. No such luck. Izzy marched past me without so much as a second look. Skye smiled at me sheepishly. Everybody, including me, knew I was in the doghouse, and I didn't have the slightest idea how I would get out of it.

While my reaction was born from pure joy, relief, happiness, and love for my daughter, I belatedly realized that having the flight attendant make an announcement was overkill. Sometimes I get caught up in a moment and take a good thing to another level. I don't regret asking the flight attendant to make that announcement, and I would absolutely do it again. In that moment, I wanted to celebrate my daughter, and this is who I am; this is how I get caught up in celebrating people I love. Thankfully, Izzy knows this about me and has long since forgiven me.

While I perhaps went a smidge too far in my show of excitement, I believe this story illustrates how much pressure both kids and parents are under during the second semester of senior year. I wish I could have genuinely believed that "it will all work out in the end," as I told Izzy during that pre-trip shopping excursion. I would have had much more fun and stressed a lot less. But clearly, I had my own set of concerns to contend with. On a side note, I'll report that Izzy was accepted to numerous colleges. *Whew!* All that worry for nothing!

When Izzy entered her freshman year at the University of Arizona, she had to report a week early for sorority recruiting. I was so nervous for her to be on her own for the first time. It was 106 degrees that week (August heat in Tucson is unrelenting), and I was petrified that she would faint or have heat stroke as she walked from house to house, chatting with the sorority girls. "Don't forget to bring your water bottle. Make sure you're wearing sunscreen. Make sure that you eat a good breakfast. Take breaks when you need them." I pummeled her with directives.

Thinking back, I realize I was projecting all my fear and worry onto her. What she probably heard was: "You have no idea how to take care of yourself, you are incapable of knowing how much food and water you need, I don't believe in you, and I'm absolutely positive you can't do life without me."

I don't know for a fact that this is what she heard, but I'm certain that I didn't convey my confidence in her ability to be on her own and "adult" while she was at school. We had to have some serious conversations during that first semester. In truth, those conversations mostly involved her asking me to sit down so she could tell me that I needed to back off and let her be. And I tried. But when I learned that this same daughter had not washed her clothes or changed her sheets in three months, I was beside myself.

"It's not your problem" was the sage advice of a good friend when I complained to her on the phone. "She will decide when she wants to do laundry, wash her clothes, and clean her sheets. Don't make this about you. It's on her to decide if and when she will do her laundry." That was hard to hear, but she was right. In month four, my daughter decided to set a weekly laundry schedule she adheres to even today.

Not all choices to let your kids figure things out independently go smoothly. And when they don't, it's not necessarily because you've done anything wrong. This is a time during which there will be lessons for both of you. You're trying to pull back and let your child "adult." Your child is trying to assert his or her independence. And you're both learning a new dance when it comes to when you swoop in and pick up the pieces when things don't go as planned versus when you step back and let your kids pick things up themselves.

I remember when Tina, a fun client, told me about the time she let her child make his own airline reservations to come home for Christmas break. "He didn't have his finals schedule yet, but he had made reservations to come home on the fifteenth of December," she recalled. "Unfortunately, his finals didn't finish until the eighteenth, and when he tried to move his reservation, because it was the busy holiday time, he couldn't get a flight home until after Christmas! My husband helped him figure out how to take the train, but it was a giant learning curve for all of us."

Depending on the age at which you decide to take a step back so your child can take a step forward, it might be helpful to keep the following in mind:

- Just because you can do it faster and more efficiently doesn't mean you should.
- Giving your children low-cost opportunities to succeed or fail gives them meaningful chances to grow and expand as human beings.
- Natural consequences are often great ways to learn lessons. For example, if your child stays up all night scrolling on their phone or playing video games and is so exhausted the next day that they don't do well on a test, maybe they won't make the same choice the next time.
- It's vital to communicate your expectations so that you both know what "adulting" looks like.

Offer space, not surveillance. Especially in the age of social media, it can be tempting to closely monitor your child's online presence. However, respecting their privacy and giving them the freedom to explore their digital spaces is crucial. Refrain from stalking them on platforms like Instagram, Facebook, TikTok, or Snapchat. Allow them to express themselves and engage with their friends in a manner separate from your watchful eye.

The more you can let go of doing everything for them and empower your children to take ownership of their lives—even before they leave home—the more you show them that you believe in their capabilities.

Letting go of trying to control every aspect of your child's life is necessary, but it's not necessarily easy. Take it slow and try to relinquish just a bit of control every day as your child inches closer to leaving home.

CHAPTER 3

Why So Far Away?

"To raise a child who is comfortable enough to leave you, means you've done your job. They are not ours to keep, but to teach how to soar on their own."
—*Anonymous*

A question that crops up regularly among my clients and friends is "Why do my kids have to go so far away?" This can apply to kids choosing to go out of state to school, enter the military, or simply move far away to pursue a new opportunity. Because it comes up so frequently, I know it's on the minds of many of you. So I want to address it early on.

Kids who leave home and move out of state (or country) generally fall into one of two categories. One, they are exceptionally confident, and they want to spread their wings and explore the world, having new and exciting experiences. Two, they want to get away from something. It could be the small town they grew up in, one they find confining. It could be past relationships or unhealthy friendships.

But it's almost *never* about trying to hurt their parents' feelings. Most kids simply don't think that way.

The majority of kids who move out of state (mine included) are open to new experiences and have a healthy sense of wonder in addition to being open to job opportunities that aren't limited to their home state. As hard as this may be for some parents who love the ability to see their kids whenever they want to, it might be precisely what a child needs to fully realize his or her potential. Of course, we don't want to stand in the way of that.

If my goal were to give you a dose of "tough love," I'd callously declare, "Snap out of it!" with a curt slap to your cheek, a la Cher in *Moonstruck*. This would be both unhelpful and hypocritical, but the intent would be to snap you back to reality, because the truth is, your child likely hasn't chosen to go far away because you did something wrong. You simply raised an independent, resourceful kid who's now pursuing his or her dreams and adulting like a boss!

I know you miss them—massively! So the question is, how do you continue to support your child and encourage them to follow their dreams while still nurturing *your* dream of having a close, connected relationship with them? The answer isn't the same for everyone, but here are some points to consider:

- Are you able to travel to see your child?
- Is your child able to come back home for a visit with some frequency?
- Are you able to help them financially so that they can visit more often?

While these questions are important, the answers don't matter until you first have a conversation with *them* to convey your desire to stay connected. It's important to note that nobody likes to feel obligated to do anything. Once a desire becomes a "should," it loses its allure. We want our kids to *want* to come home, not feel as though they have to.

When we talk about how having them home under one roof—whether for a night or a week—makes us feel complete, happy, peaceful, or content, we have to remember that until they have kids of their own, those explanations may be a stretch for them to truly understand. To help them better understand your perspective, you could liken it to "getting the band back together." You know, those nights when their best friends from high school come over and they talk into the night, tell stories, reminisce, and feel like nobody knows them better. Let them know that's what it feels like to have them home.

And (there's always an "and") we don't get to make our kids do anything. We can have important conversations and tell them our thoughts and desires while also (perhaps more importantly) listening to *their* thoughts and desires.

You of course don't want to bully, manipulate, coerce, or guilt your kids into spending more time with you than they're comfortable spending. You want them to *want* to spend that time with you. And if they don't want that right now (remember, you don't know what the future holds), you have a choice. You can make it mean that they don't love (or even like) you anymore and want to be as far away as possible, or you can make it mean that they are simply exerting their right to create their own life as they see fit. Maybe it's a job, a girl, a boy, a new city, a new country, or a new experience altogether that's calling them away. But in my experience, it's best to support their decisions (unless they are harmful) and give them our blessing to go, do, and be the best versions of themselves while reminding them that wherever they are, we love them, support them, and want only the best for them.

WAYS TO SURVIVE A LONG-DISTANCE RELATIONSHIP WITH ADULT CHILDREN

Set Up a Time to Chat
My friend Carrie set up a time to talk with her son on Sundays at 4PM. (Take note of the suggestion in chapter 11 regarding flexibility when it comes to scheduled chats.)

Make Plans to Get Together

It's always nice to have something on the calendar to look forward to.

Try to Keep Old Traditions Going

Continue to look forward to the Fourth of July BBQ, family Thanksgiving, and birthday gatherings, with the caveat that things change and the understanding that your kids may not be able to attend these events every year, depending on their schedules.

Create New Traditions

Ask your kids what works for them. Try to be creative, and focus on fun, not being too stringent in your expectations.

Have an Open Mindset

Being in the moment, flexible, and easy-going will attract more positive end results than having a fixed mindset of how things "ought to be." I know it doesn't always work out the way you imagine, and it can hurt when it doesn't. Reality doesn't always fit your "ideal" vision. After all, aren't all your kids supposed to grow up and buy homes on the same cul-de-sac as you? Every morning, you'll sit on one of your front porches, sharing a blueberry scone while sipping frothy lattes. I saw those Hallmark movies too, but I have yet to see that dynamic play out in real life. So make your own Hallmark magic. Be present during the time you do have with your kids, and get on with creating your own beautiful life.

∽

Here's the truth and the core reason it's so essential to make peace with your child choosing a college or after-high-school destination that's not within close proximity: It might not be a temporary choice.

Many times, after graduating from college, kids choose not to move back to their hometowns. This happens for a variety of reasons. Sometimes they have better job prospects in bigger cities, or they decide they want to explore the world a bit more. Often, it's a combination of reasons. Perhaps staying in their college town is easier, they want to continue to live near their friends, or they simply decide that moving home is too much work.

It's usually *not* any of the reasons moms initially fear: "They don't love me anymore," "They don't want to be close to family," or "They are rejecting their upbringing." I promise you, it's quite seldom that our adult kids put that much thought into it.

The real question is, what do you do with your broken heart and your unrealized expectations? You have several options, but only one of them will bring you the result you want (and no, it's not your kid moving back home). It's identifying a way to feel better about the fact that they aren't moving home.

I've got good news and bad news. Let's address the bad news, which you likely already know: We cannot control other people. I know, I know. I hate it too! I have *so* many people I'd like to have under my control, not just my hubby, daughter, mother, sister, and boss (wait, I am the boss!).

Now for the good news: You are the boss of you! That means that you are entirely responsible for your happiness. Admittedly, it took me a while to get on board with this concept, and it might take you a minute as well.

"Don't my kids affect my ability to be happy, Allie?" Yes and no. Let me explain.

Many parents (especially devoted mothers) seem to ride a rollercoaster of emotions when it comes to their kids. What's the saying: "You're only as happy as your most unhappy child"? That's great for those of us who only have one child (assuming he or she is happy), but it only holds true if you allow yourself to be enmeshed with your kids in such a way that you no longer have a sense of self, and you've merged your identity and emotional well-being with that of your kids. Yes, this was me. That's how I know. Again, why didn't they give us the complete user manual when we gave birth to these kids?

The key to accepting many of our adult kids' decisions is realizing that resisting "what is" will not bring us what we want. The more we can lean in, get curious, and, yes, even accept these unwelcome choices, the more we will set ourselves up for a better and more connected relationship with our adult kids.

CHAPTER 4

Step One: Be Good to Yourself

"It is so important for you to take time for yourself and find clarity. The most important relationship is the one you have with yourself."
—*Diane von Fursternberg*

I love gardening. Or maybe I should say, I love fresh flowers, homegrown vegetables, and the *idea* that when I plant some seeds, a few months later I'll reap a beautiful bounty. While gardening and sowing seeds are grossly overused as metaphors, hang with me, because if you're also a visual person, it's hard to come up with an alternative that makes nearly as much sense when it comes to nurturing ourselves.

Before we get into the answer to "Now What?" that surely played a huge part in you picking up this book, I want to address the ways in which we nurture ourselves and how important a role that plays in our overall happiness. The way we nurture our thoughts and our bodies affects how we show up, how we take action, and ultimately, how we feel about our lives.

As I'm writing this, my beloved island of Maui has just suffered catastrophic fires that completely wiped out the town of Lahaina and affected the nearby areas of Kula and Kihei. I went into a trance similar to the one I went into after September 11, 2001, watching videos and footage nonstop for an entire week. I was unable to fully comprehend the loss of life, loss of homes, and overall effect on the culture of such a magical place.

Unfortunately, this kind of news isn't uncommon these days. From mass shootings, horrific murders, wars, and the general dismantling of humanity, it's all on display daily if you choose to look for it.

I've learned the hard way that, because I'm a sensitive person, it does not behoove me to take in daily tragedies. I like to keep lightly informed and only delve deep into crises, such as the fires in Maui, when they not only affect me personally but also affect those I know and love.

All of this to say that while you are in this new, empty-nest phase of life, make sure that you are being intentional when it comes to what you allow into your life. In the last few years, I have been extremely intentional about editing out toxic friends and energy vampires. I also try not to consume any more bad news than necessary—or at least even it out with positive stories and optimistic viewpoints. This is your one and only life. Make sure you take great care of yourself mentally, physically, and emotionally.

This seems like as good a time as any to introduce a self-coaching concept that has significantly impacted my life and my clients' lives. It has to do with how we view circumstances that occur and, as a result, how we approach those circumstances. When coaching, I often use this model to help my clients see how their thoughts directly affect their feelings and, in turn, inspire their actions.

I'll first explain the concept, then give you some examples so you can see how it plays out in real life. After that, I'll give you an opportunity to practice it.

CTFAR SELF-COACHING MODEL

C = Circumstance

A circumstance is a neutral fact that all would agree upon. For example, "It's Monday." We're not talking about subjective experiences ("Mondays stink"). At the most basic level, a circumstance could be that the sun came out today. What's important to recognize is that, on their own, circumstances are neutral—they aren't good or bad, right or wrong. Until, that is, we give them meaning. It always helps me to remember that circumstances never include adjectives.

T = Thought

A thought is a sentence or phrase that comes to mind about a particular circumstance. For example, "I'm so glad the sun is out today. I've been wanting to take a walk." Or "Shoot, the sun is out today. I'm so tired of 100-degree days."

F = Feeling

A feeling is a sensation in our body that occurs as a result of the thoughts we have. If you're excited about the sun being out, you might feel joyful. If you're frustrated that the sun is out, you may feel annoyed.

A = Action

Action is what we do and don't do in response to our thoughts and feelings. Keeping with our sunny day example, if you're happy about the sun and feeling joyful, you may jump out of bed and attack the day. If you're disappointed with the sunny day, you might roll over and go back to sleep.

R = Result

The result is what does (and doesn't) happen due to the above series of events. If you're happy, you'll go for a walk and enjoy the morning. If you're unhappy, you'll stay in bed and get nothing done. What's important is to see how the end result is driven by the initial thought you had about a neutral circumstance.

Here is a more specific example that empty-nest

moms might be able to relate to.

C = Drop-off day at college
T = "I am not ready for them to leave" *versus* "I am so proud!"
F = Worried/fearful *versus* confident
A = Clings tightly and acts nervous *versus* empowers child and projects confidence
R = Mom is stuck in worry and fear and can't enjoy the day *versus* mom is confident in the kid's capabilities and her own capabilities to be okay.

To add another example, if the circumstance is "My child is leaving home next week," and I think the thought, "I am capable and I can do anything I put my mind to" over and over again, it will become deeply rooted in my mind and become a *belief*—a thought which appears to be fact.

On the other hand, if I think the thought, "I have no idea what to do with the rest of my life" over and over again, I will start to believe *that* to be true. When any thought goes unchecked, we begin to believe it to be true. So let's focus on ensuring that our thoughts are the ones we *want* to be true!

What's most important to remember is that just because we think something doesn't make it true. Again, *thoughts are not facts.* That idea seems obvious on paper, but it's harder to recognize in moment-to-moment life. Just because I think I hear a noise in the middle of the night does not mean that there is indeed a robber trying to break into my house. It only means I had a thought (words in my brain); it's not verified truth.

On any given day, we have between 60,000 and 85,000 thoughts, and most of these thoughts are both repetitive and subconscious. One way to determine which thoughts you're choosing "on purpose" is to do a "brain drain" or thought download. Don't worry, this isn't as complicated (or messy) as it sounds. Simply grab a pen and a piece of paper and write down everything you're thinking. Doing this first thing in the morning often works best, as you aren't entirely conscious and therefore aren't judging your thoughts as much as you might later in the day.

An example of a "brain drain":

"I hate waking up early in the morning. It's so cold out. I don't want to get out of bed, but I need to because I said I'd go with my friend to work out. Why did I make that commitment? Why so early? I don't know. I'll be fine once I get there. I do love yoga. And I'm looking forward to seeing my friend."

Basically, it's stream-of-consciousness writing.

If we take the above example and circle thoughts that seem positive, helpful, and perhaps motivating, we will circle "*I'll be fine once I get there,*" "*I love yoga,*" and "*I'm looking forward to seeing my friend.*"

If we choose to focus on those thoughts, they might produce feelings such as **determination**, **connection**, and **joy**. These feelings will help provide the fuel necessary to motivate us to meet our friends and enjoy our morning yoga session together.

However, if I didn't consciously focus on the thoughts that I felt would serve me better and instead focused on "*I hate waking up early,*" "*I don't want to get out of bed,*" and "*Why did I make this commitment?*" I might have feelings of **resentment**, **frustration**, or **anger**. Those feelings would more than likely produce actions such as rolling over and going back to sleep, not meeting my friend, and not working out. As a result, they'd more than likely contribute to feeling disappointed in myself later on.

Isn't that amazing? Nothing changed except the thoughts I focused on! If you want to learn more about this, you can delve deeper into the self-coaching model, which I learned from Brooke Castillo through the Life Coach School.

Now it's your turn. Choose a challenging issue you're having trouble with, and use the self-coaching model to identify the five aspects of how you're getting from circumstance to result and how you might be able to alter your thoughts to alter the end result.

C
T
F
A
R

Just as your mindset is critical when it comes to being intentional about how you want to feel, so is the way you care for your physical body. Although none of the below suggestions are particularly new or earth-shattering, my clients and I have found that when practiced consistently, they make a noticeable impact on our quality of life and well-being.

As with all the suggestions in this book, take what works for you and leave the rest. There is no one-size-fits-all recipe for how to create your ideal life.

SIMPLE, HIGHLY IMPACTFUL PRACTICES WHEN ENTERING YOUR EMPTY-NEST YEARS

I'm going to assume that you are aware of four of the oft-mentioned "basics of well-being": meditation, hydration, exercise, and sleep. I'm also going to bet that you could benefit from a reminder, because the minute we get stressed, overwhelmed, and busy, the first things we forget are the basics. If you're like me, unless you're in dire pain or experiencing a health crisis, you can easily forget to do the simplest things that can significantly impact your life. So let's review.

Meditation
Don't worry, this isn't the scary sit-on-your-cushion-for-an-hour kind of meditation that may come to mind when you hear the word. The very thought of that

makes me antsy! I'm suggesting as few as five minutes a day. If you can commit to taking five minutes first thing in the morning to ground yourself and breathe for thirty days straight, I promise you will see results.

When we take time to become fully present and tap into a universal energy, we open the door to divine inspiration, wisdom, and clarity. Who doesn't want that? I have found, both for myself and for my clients, that this simple act of pausing first thing in the morning sets up the day with greater intention, allowing for more ease and flow throughout.

My favorite meditation apps are *Calm, Headspace, MindValley, and Gabby* (Gabby Bernstein's app). I use one for a few months and then switch it up so I don't get bored. On a practical level, have your App downloaded beforehand and your AirPods charged and ready to go. Sometimes I make a cup of tea, light a candle, sit up straight in a chair, and pretend I am an enlightened being. Other times I pop in my AirPods while lying horizontal in bed, next to my sleeping husband. Whatever works. As Nike says, "Just do it."

Hydration

The human body is made up of about sixty percent water. If you aren't properly hydrated, you won't think properly, move with ease, digest easily, or eliminate waste efficiently. I am not a natural-born water drinker. Like exercise, I had to trick myself into making this basic task easier.

In contrast to water, I *love* tea. So to help myself stay hydrated, I prepare a large pot of tea every morning. I also make protein shakes with water and make "spa water" in a pretty pitcher. If I'm going to be at my desk all day working, I bring in a tray with four different drinks: tea, water, a shake, and sometimes Diet Coke (I know, I know). I have found that if I prepare all of these options ahead of time, over the course of a few hours I will consume them all. But if I don't, I often forget to take even a sip of water all day! Just know that when you're well-hydrated, you think, move, and act better. The End.

Exercise

The word alone can be triggering for some people. If you're not doing it, you might experience shame. To avoid that, let's change the word from "exercise" to "movement." Honestly, if you can move your body in a way that is both comfortable and pleasurable, you'll do it more often *and* enjoy it more.

Find an activity you enjoy and simply commit to moving your body every day. I'm not suggesting you train for a marathon or sign up for a weightlifting competition (though if you do, amazing!). I'm simply suggesting that you find a way to move your body consistently for at least thirty minutes every day. It's okay if you're not sporty or haven't been one to engage in activities such as tennis, golf, or running. Simply walking for thirty minutes a day at a semi-brisk pace will yield increased dopamine, heightened metabolism, and an overall feeling of well-being. Plus, you don't need to worry about equipment or schedules!

If possible, walking outdoors gives you the added benefit of getting some valuable vitamin D and connecting with nature. As I mentioned, I had to trick myself into exercising on the regular. Laying out my attire, shoes, socks, hat, and glasses the night before was key to ensuring that I actually went on my walk.

Calling a friend to create a walking appointment is another excellent way to ensure that you will show up. Plus, you get the benefit of connection. If you are more adventuresome and physically fit, I encourage you to look into other fun ways to move your body. My current favorites are Pickleball, paddle boarding, surfing, hiking, and weight training. I'm working on liking yoga, Pilates, and anything that stretches my poor muscles. And I highly encourage massages whenever possible!

Sleep

Like exercise, sleep can be a dirty word, so let's refer to this basic need as "rest." The issue with sleep typically isn't that we aren't doing it. It's that we aren't getting enough of it or getting it at a high enough quality.

If we don't get enough rest, we aren't able to show up as our best selves. As I write this, I have only been sleeping for five hours each night—far less than the optimal seven to nine hours my body requires. But I've been traveling and am therefore jet-lagged. I know that over the course of the next week, I will sleep when I can and rest when I feel compelled to do so. As extremely busy moms, we often don't recognize our body's signals to rest. But as empty-nest moms, we have an opportunity to retrain our bodies and brains to pay attention to our natural sleep and wake cycles.

The older I get, the more I like to wake up early, which, as a lifelong night owl, is weird and wonderful! Most of my clients report that they too have enjoyed getting up earlier, engaging in their newfound morning routine, and retiring earlier in the evening. I used to think this meant we were old, but now I know it means we are smart!

∼

Paying attention to our thoughts is such a simple (although not necessarily easy) way to get an accurate reading of self-talk and, in turn, our mindset. If we notice that we are habitually focusing on what isn't working in our lives without balancing it with what is working, we will probably believe that our life is in the dumps! It's far more likely that some things that are going well while a few "noisy" things are not (yet) up to par. The key is to give equal airtime to both sides. And, as mentioned above, focus on and be grateful for the things that *are* working.

Attuning to both our mind and body, especially when we are feeling any type of loss or sadness, is vital. When we make time and space for ourselves (by this point, you know I am going to suggest you prioritize *your* needs), we allow our feelings to pass through us. This frees us up to get creative, innovative, and open to the myriad possibilities life will offer.

Focusing on self-care may feel too indulgent at first, but think of your body like a car and make sure you keep up with the maintenance. Oil changes equal doctor appointments, refilling your tank equals proper nutrition and sufficient sleep, and rotating your tires equals a massage or perhaps a chiropractic adjustment. When approached that way, how fun does it become? The bottom line is, the better you care for your body, mind, soul (and car), the better they will perform and the more mileage you'll get from them.

CHAPTER 5

The Truth About Who You Are (and Who You'll Become)

"She said 'I'm not giving up. The woman I'll be a few years from now is counting on me.' And the world shifted."
—*Nakeia Homer*

Because we've been conditioned to believe that all the "doing" we've done as moms is simply what we should do, we often discount the laundry list of tasks we've completed over the years to make our family members' lives easier. It's as though completing the daily to-do-for-family list is simply a given, an automatic responsibility that's as required as a car seat and a package of diapers to bring the baby home. We don't tend to consider the notion that we had a choice in the matter. But we did then, and we do now.

Beyond evaluating (or re-evaluating) your mindset and recommitting to solid self-care practices, it's important to acknowledge how far you've come and what you've accomplished so you can remind yourself of how capable you truly are of moving toward an incredible empty-nest life.

In case you need a bit of help remembering, let's begin with the most basic yet frequently unacknowledged accomplishments from the past eighteen years, starting with meal prep. If you made just one child's lunches from first through eighth grade, that's approximately 1,440 lunches. In some places, that qualifies you as a chef! You attended at least sixteen parent/teacher conferences, supervised homework for ten to fifteen years, organized and hosted eighteen birthday parties, and let's not even get into how many sports practices, games, extracurricular activities, and school-sanctioned events you either attended or were responsible for organizing. All of this puts you on par with the organizers of the Olympics. Or NATO. Speaking of NATO, you have most likely refereed hundreds of arguments, sidestepped numerous potential booby-traps, and dealt with countless how-do-we-handle-this situations over the last two decades. Why are you not running for president, being offered the secretary of state position, or working at the Department of Defense?

My point is, the skill sets you've developed (one

meal and negotiation at a time) and the accomplishments you've had over these many years are nothing short of remarkable. Now is the time for you to reflect on all your behind-the-scenes wins to see what a truly impressive mother you are, while reminding yourself that you can once again apply that level of focus to achieve whatever you set your sights on.

To that end, in this chapter we'll explore the areas of your life where you feel you've made a difference and feel purposeful. Taking the time to reflect on your wins and accomplishments not only reminds you of your capabilities but often is the springboard to summoning the necessary confidence to try new experiences.

Please take the time to do the following exercise.

ACCOMPLISHMENT INVENTORY EXERCISE

List 5 Things You're Proud of Accomplishing
Example:
1. I raised 4 kids.
2. I volunteered at the hospital.
3. I helped with school fundraisers.
4. I received a pay raise at work.
5. I stayed married, even when it was (really) hard.

List 5 Things You're Known For

Example:

1. Planning and organization skills
2. Kindness and empathy
3. Making delicious cookies
4. Good listener
5. Not a gossip

List 5 Things Your Kids Would Say They Love About You

Example:

1. They can count on my support.
2. I know how to make them feel loved.
3. I'm amazing at throwing together a dinner for a crowd.
4. The way I always seem to have what they need in my purse.
5. The way I love to go to their games and cheer them on.

List 5 Things Your Spouse/Best Friend/Partner Would Say About You

Example:

1. I take care of everybody's needs first.
2. I am an exceptional wife/mother/daughter/friend.
3. I know just how to make a house feel warm and inviting.
4. I am endlessly supportive of other's dreams.

5. I sometimes forget to take care of myself.

Whether you realize it or not, through this exercise you're already creating the beginning of your roadmap to an incredible empty-nest life. When you can notice where you are now and where you've been, it removes the tendency to focus on where you *should* be going and instead allows you to concentrate on where you *want* to go. It's step one on your journey to intentionally creating the person you want to be and the life you'd like to have from this point forward.

It is critical during this life transition not to compare yourself or your journey with others' journey, even that of your closest friends. The way we deal with change is largely determined by our past, our expectations, our desires, and our thoughts on how things "should be." Just as each child is different, your empty-nest life journey will be different (possibly completely different) than that of your best friend, sister, or cousin.

A number of my clients have gotten stuck in the "compare and despair" cycle. Jessie told me, "Linda and I have daughters the same age, and they have done everything together. They both left for college simultaneously, and when I look at Linda, it's like life didn't skip a beat. She's traveling all over with her hubby, she took up Pickleball, and she has a side hustle selling a skincare system. Linda loved being a mom, but it looks like she's loving this part of her life as much, if not more, while I'm floundering. I have no idea what I want to do for the next twenty to thirty years besides be a grandparent. I feel like such a loser and so out of step with my life. What's wrong with me?"

If you're feeling like Jessie, struggling with day-to-day life and uncertain about the future, like you're stuck in a holding pattern, you are like ninety-five percent of my clients! It's normal not to know exactly what you want the next chapter of life to look like. That's why it's so important to take some time to refocus your attention on your own wants and desires. And this is where we can start to look at not only who we've been, but who we get to become.

So many women I talk with have no idea what they like and don't like anymore. Most moms can barely remember life before kids, so why are we surprised that it takes a period of adjustment to get to know the current version of ourselves?

When Connie came to me, she said she had no idea who she was if she wasn't a full-time mom. "It's all I ever wanted to be, and now I feel like the thing I'm best at has been taken away. It's embarrassing, but I don't know who I am if I'm not a mom."

I asked her if she was willing to play a little game with me. I'd ask her some simple questions, and we'd go from there. I asked questions like "Are you a morning or evening person?" "Do you like coffee or tea?" "Do you prefer to take baths or showers?" She looked at me with a worried expression and replied, "I have no idea. Besides knowing I don't like coffee, I have always done whatever was quickest and most efficient for the family. I never really thought about what I liked."

I gave Connie some homework. Each day, she had to ask herself, "What do I *feel* like today?" I emphasize the word *feel* because your body is the best barometer to determine what you like and what you don't like. Your barometer is your internal compass, and it will give you an accurate reading—*if* you take the time to tune into it.

Each day, Connie was to ask herself "What do I feel like doing, eating, drinking, seeing, being today?" And then, she was to try out each choice like she was trying on a new blouse and ask herself the following questions: "How does this 'blouse' make me feel? Do I like the color, the fit, the texture?" She came back the next week and reported that she was, in fact, a morning person. "I used to stay up late, waiting on the kids, but I hated it. I was always so tired; I felt like I was going against my natural bodily rhythm. Now I wake up early and I love the silence before the day gets started. I had no idea!"

I asked Connie about what she figured out for the rest of the day, and she told me that this was still a work in progress. "Some days I like to go for a walk, and some days I feel like volunteering at the church. I just keep trying new things and then make a note of what makes me feel good and what doesn't."

The opposite of tuning in to our own internal

guidance system is what I call "canvassing the committee." Typically, it occurs when you have to make a decision, and rather than tuning in to your own innate wisdom, you ask your group of friends what they think. "Should I call and check on her? Should I drive up there and surprise him? Should I cut bangs?" It's something I used to do all the time when I was a new mother and wasn't confident making decisions for my young baby by myself.

It makes sense that when you haven't fully developed self-trust and a belief in your own personal self-knowing, you will feel more comfortable polling others whom you trust rather than relying on your own opinion.

The process of trying on new things can work for you too.

EXERCISE

10 Things I'd Like to Try

Example:

1. Yoga class
2. Açaí Bowl
3. Meditation
4. Knitting
5. Bird watching
6. Pickleball
7. Pottery class
8. Cross-country skiing

9. Pilates
10. Puppet making

Commit to trying one item or activity each week. The best way to make this happen is to schedule it. Put it on your calendar, and "obey the calendar." I find that if it's on my calendar, it's a commitment, so I do it. No excuses. The key is to pay attention to how each new activity (or food) makes you feel. Does it make you feel energized? Joyful? Content? Drained?

Keep this list going for the next few months. Ideally, your days will begin to include more items that are inspiring, energizing, and uplifting as time goes on. You want to minimize as many draining and depleting activities as possible. Approaching your days in this way will help you develop a deeper trust in yourself and help you navigate paths you have yet to explore with clarity and confidence.

I find this approach quite empowering, but a few of my clients don't like it…at first. I remember Linda initially telling me she hated the thought that she was entirely responsible for her choices and her life. "It makes me feel like I have so much pressure to get it 100 percent right. If I don't, I've failed myself."

I told her I understood and asked if she was willing to consider a thought reframe. "What if you *are* 100 percent responsible, meaning that your life, at this present moment, is the result of each and every decision you have made up to this point? Life didn't just 'happen to you'; you created the life you are living. So if you don't like your current circumstances—your home, your job, or your attitude—*you*, and you alone, have the power to change it."

After that, Linda found this exercise both exciting and scary. "I like the idea of having control, but I need to make friends with the idea of taking total responsibility for my life. I think blaming others or things that didn't go my way was just an excuse. Now I see that I have the power to create what I want and don't have to wait for someone or something to come save me!"

It's true, you don't need to rely on anyone else. In fact, you truly *can't* count on anyone else to make you happy or make you feel a certain way anyway. I find that fact *very* empowering!

So go ahead and dream and scheme. Looking at the lists above, go ahead and decide. Choose one thing that you want to focus on. Don't worry, you can always choose again. But for the first step, you just need to get a little momentum. Try one new thing for one week.

CHAPTER 6

So…Now What?!

"Be open to what comes next for you. You may be heading in one direction and then life brings you another that might be a good thing."
—*Natalie Cane*

I often wonder how many moms give a significant amount of thought to their life post-kids before their kids move out. I gave it nearly none, and most moms I talk to have also been so kid-focused for the previous many years that "the empty-nest" phase arrives with a bit of a sudden shock when, on the first morning of this new life, you don't have to wake to an alarm or orchestrate your day around drop-off, pick-up, sports practices, and meals. This can be oddly unnerving. The whole day (and then the whole week) looms ahead with no structure, no one to attend to, and little if any idea of what to do with oneself.

If what I've just described sounds familiar, please know that what you're feeling is extremely common. When you're having a mini-freak-out session and asking yourself, "Now What?!" you're in good company. Let's unpack it.

I find that it's best to answer the question "Now what?" in bite-size pieces, because honestly, who knows *exactly* what they want to do after being a full-time mom for so long? If you are one of the few who do, bravo! If you're like the rest of us and only started easing your way into thinking about what you want to do next at the end of the last chapter, grab a journal and a pen, and let's go about this as though you are a combo of Nancy Drew and the Dalai Lama.

The goal is to lead with curiosity while maintaining a certain amount of detachment as you go through this process. Think of it like shopping a sample sale. While you might feel the need to grab everything and throw it in your basket, if you take the time to sift underneath piles, you may locate a hidden gem. In approaching it in this way, you will almost certainly be further along than the person who fills up their basket out of fear of missing out on something they probably didn't like or need.

I love a good metaphor (if you couldn't already tell), and for this practice, I encourage you to embark upon it as though you're going on a journey. I know, a minute ago you were a combo of Nancy Drew and the Dalai Lama, but let's add in Dora the Explorer, just for fun.

As a travel buff, one thing I know for sure is that when I'm embarking on a road trip, I never want to just jump in a car and start driving. At a minimum, I must first decide whether I want to head towards the beach or the mountains. If it's the latter, will I be needing snow tires? What are all the fun sights that I can stop and admire along the way?

This next chapter of your life is *your* journey, and you get to design it exactly the way you'd like. While you may have given a good bit of thought to your starting point (Empty-Nest Land), make no mistake: this journey is less about reaching an über-specific destination and far more about who you intend to *become* during the process.

Having fun with this planning process makes for a far more enjoyable experience overall, so as you begin the adventure of creating your next chapter as an empty nester, attempt to bring the same energy you would bring when planning a bucket-list trip to Hawaii or Europe or Africa. Think of all the things you would like to do and see. Consider who you will need to become to navigate the journey safely and successfully (and with loads of laughter and good snacks)! The more time you put into considering exactly what it is you want, the higher the chances that you will be successful in creating the life that you want and deserve.

Let's first take some time to consider exactly where it is you want to go. In other words, which aspects of your life are you completely content with, and which aspects would you like to change a bit now that life is shifting? To clarify, you don't have to start *completely* from scratch. If there are some aspects of or activities from your "previous" life, such as working out, book club, or cooking gourmet meals a few nights a week that you'd like to continue, fantastic! This is the time to Marie Kondo what's in your life today in order to assess what stays and what goes.

To decide how to refocus your time and attention, it's a good idea first to identify what is important to you now. This may be a bit challenging, since for the last couple of decades, everything you deemed important was seen through the lens of being a parent. But guess what: it now gets to be based solely on what feels good to *you*!

Many years ago, I learned about "Desire Mapping" from Danielle LaPorte. Desire Mapping is the process of identifying your values—or Core Desired Feelings (CDFs)—and then creating your life based on how you want to feel. (If you can't already tell, we'll be revisiting the importance of noticing how things make you *feel* a lot when it comes to designing your next chapter.) The purpose of taking the time to identify your CDFs and your intrinsic values is that it allows you to recognize the power you have to create your life. When we listen to our guidance system, which is always giving us clues as to what our CDFs are, we can make empowered decisions that will help create an ideal life based on how we want to feel (because obviously, you don't want to continue to feel directionless, lonely, or otherwise untethered!).

Identifying your core desired feelings is necessary before you can know where to put your energy and attention in the coming years to create your ideal next chapter of life. Here is a quick exercise to get you started:

Ask yourself the following questions:

- How do I want to feel when I first wake up in the morning?
- How do I want to feel when I look at my calendar or to-do list?
- How do I want to feel when I set a goal or go after a dream?
- How do I want to feel when I think about getting together with my family or friends?

I remember when Jamie told me that she "just wants to feel happy again." I nodded my head, because ninety-eight percent of people, when asked "How do you want to feel?" respond with "happy!" But what does "happy" really mean? Not in debt? Madly in love with your spouse? Physically healthy? Feeling happy looks different to different people, so it's important to figure out what "happy" looks like—and, most importantly, feels like—for you.

To dive a bit deeper into her definition of "happy," I asked Jamie to tell me what happy *feels* like to her. She said she wanted to feel light and joyful again. "I loved being a full-time mom and made sure that, as a family, we had a lot of fun times together. But now that the kids are gone, I don't feel like I have that built-in opportunity to laugh and be silly." That was such great insight! When prompted, Jamie could easily identify where in her life she feels joyful and light (and maybe even a little silly): when she's hanging out with her kids. "You know, my husband and I used to go to the comedy club before we had kids. I loved that! Also, sometimes when I am with my girlfriends and we're just hanging out on the back patio, having some wine and just laughing about funny things we've done, that brings me joy."

Great! She identified two core desired feelings: *light* and *joyful*. And she recognized that when she's with her girlfriends or watching comedy with her hubby, she feels those feelings. So now, the trick was to find other activities and ways for her to spend her time that also create those feelings of being light and joyful.

Beyond more general words like happy, excited, or motivated, how *else* do you want to feel? Circle 8-10 adjectives from the following list that describe how you'd like to feel day-in and day-out (or choose your own feeling words):

Courageous	Relaxed	Fulfilled	Inspired
Peaceful	Open Free	Excited	Happy
Delighted	Joyful	Content	Vibrant
Calm	Passionate	Adventurous	Safe
Refreshed	Accepting	Powerful	Proud
Caring	Confident	Connected	Strong
Loving	Curious	Playful	Creative
Grounded	Determined	Present	Brave

Now, edit your list down to three or four words. These are the words that resonate most with your soul and the feelings you want to generate and cultivate on a daily basis. The way you do that is by purposely designing your days with these feelings in mind.

When I first discovered the desire mapping process in 2015, my desired feelings were: divinely connected, creatively inspired, vibrantly healthy, and anchored in ease. Nearly ten years later, these are still my core desired feelings. I've also added empowered, free, and blessed.

For me to feel vibrantly healthy, I know I need to get at least seven hours of sleep, drink lots of water, exercise or move my body for an hour a day, and meditate and practice gratitude. So when I look at my plans for each day, I ensure I've included each of these activities.

Monica's CDFs are useful, loved, and appreciated. Monica is an empty-nest mom as well as a speech therapist. She told me that her work—helping students with their speech—makes her feel useful. Her relationship with her kids, husband, and parents helps her to feel loved. And her volunteer work in her church gives her a feeling of being appreciated.

The more specific you can get when identifying with your unique CDFs, the more clarity you will have, not only in setting goals and organizing your calendar but also in determining who you want to spend time with and who you don't.

For example, Julie told me that when she is at work, she feels powerless, disrespected, and on edge all the time. When we assessed her CDFs, we determined them to be independent, joyful, and free. Since those feelings don't align with how she feels at work, and she cannot change her work environment or the way her boss treats her, she realized that she should probably look for a new job.

Paying attention to how you feel in daily life as a result of your interactions and activities gives you powerful information to determine whether you feel aligned with your CDFs or things feel askew.

Take a look at your calendar for the next couple of months. Review your schedule, including your appointments, events, and obligations. Take a moment to check in with your body and examine how you feel about these commitments. For example, if you are scheduled to go to lunch with an old—but no longer close—friend, and the feeling of dread comes up when you consider that date, you might want to reconsider whether the lunch date is in your best interests.

Similarly, if you have a bunch of "have to dos" on your list, such as dentist or doctor appointments, filing taxes, or a weekend at your in-laws, and you know that you can't cancel any of these activities, you can instead choose to feel (insert one of your CDFs) by exploring your thoughts about each activity and consciously choosing to focus on the positive. Perhaps you will feel relieved or satisfied to have honored your commitment. The point is, you are in charge of your life. You can't always choose your circumstances or what happens to you in life, but you can choose how you react to it and feel about it.

Consider those moments when you're stuck in traffic. Perhaps you feel frustrated, angry, and upset because you're running late. Alternatively, you could use this as an opportunity to listen to a podcast, make a quick phone call, or listen to upbeat music. Your circumstances don't have to change in the least, but your reaction to them is ultimately your choice. Taking the time to identify and use your CDFs to create your day-to-day life will help create a life where you feel more aligned with your true core values and priorities.

CHAPTER 7

Is It Time to Get a Cat?

"Loneliness is proof that your innate search for connection is intact."
−Martha Beck

Now that you're feeling more empowered about the level of control you have over the roadmap that will take you into this next phase of your life, let's address one of the most common feelings moms have when their final (or only) kid leaves home: loneliness.

It can be a hard pill to swallow that we're surrounded by family and friends, yet we still feel exceptionally lonely. One of the reasons this occurs is that while we aren't physically alone, we feel alone in our experience. Additionally, perhaps we are unwilling to be vulnerable enough to share our feelings with others.

When our daughter left for college, I remember feeling certain nobody had ever felt the way I was feeling. Although it's true that we all have unique experiences, the feeling of isolation—compounded by the embarrassment and shame I felt because I was having difficulty adjusting—created a heightened feeling of loneliness for me.

A common solution to "I'm lonely" seems to be getting a pet. This is true for both men and women, and it's certainly not unique to those experiencing an empty nest. The notion of getting a cat or a dog when the kids leave is not, on the surface, a terrible idea. The space that is left when our kids leave needs to be filled. The trick is filling it with the right thing (nachos, margaritas, ice cream, and potato chips sound—and are—good fillers initially, but that lifestyle isn't sustainable!).

Now, to be clear, I think cats are lovely. And while several of my best friends have cats, I am, and will most likely always be, a dog mom. That being said, it really doesn't matter whether you are considering a dog, a cat, a hamster, or an iguana; what's important is knowing why you think you suddenly need a pet (or another pet, if your house already runneth over in this area).

If you've had a busy household for the last many years and now your house seems too quiet, with nothing clamoring for your attention, perhaps now actually is a good time to look into getting a new pet. But if you have never owned a dog, suddenly bringing home a high-energy Goldendoodle with thoughts of it being your new companion, making you feel less lonely and more needed, is an action you might want to think twice about.

My friend (let's call her Lisa so as not to publicly puppy-shame her) adopted a miniature dachshund from the Denver Dumb Friends League a month after her twin boys went to college. She thought all her extra time would go toward loving and training this adorable pup. Aptly named Rascal, he had other ideas. Yes, he was cute and cuddly, but he also had a fondness for eating underwear or anything else left on the floor. He refused to be potty trained, and when he wasn't peeing in the kitchen (while making direct eye contact with Lisa), he would sneak off to the living room and do his other business in private, behind the coach. This led to a mysterious odor that only became obvious when the stench became so vile that she couldn't focus on watching her beloved "Yellowstone" at night with her hubby.

Eventually, Lisa realized that she and Rascal needed help. After three months of intensive boot camp (which they both had to attend), Rascal learned the basics, and Lisa learned to set better boundaries. When I asked Lisa if she would recommend getting a puppy to other empty nesters, she said, "Maybe a goldfish or a dog that's already been trained and whose family moved away. I think it would have been nice to have a dog who was missing his family like I was missing my boys."

Acquiring a new pet is certainly one way to combat loneliness. But taking the time to look at where the loneliness actually stems from is often far more helpful. Certainly, you're missing your child. I didn't only miss having our daughter around; I also missed feeling needed. I hadn't realized how much I'd relied on the sense of being needed on the daily.

You've probably heard the adage "A woman can be in a room full of people and still feel lonely." Loneliness is a feeling. And it's different from "I have too much time on my hands," which is a thought one has based on a feeling (I'll talk more about the thought "I have too much time on my hands" in the next chapter). It's also different from "I don't feel connected to anyone" (which I'll address in chapter 9).

If you are feeling a sense of loneliness, now might be a good time to dive a little deeper and see what's underneath that initial feeling.

Ask yourself the following questions:
- When do I feel lonely? What time of day is this feeling most common?
- When I feel lonely, what are my thoughts?
- Do I believe that the empty nest is what is causing my feelings of loneliness?
- If my kids came home today, would I automatically not feel lonely anymore?
- Do I feel like my kids provide my most natural sense of being connected to others?

- Is there a possibility that, even with the kids not at home, I can make meaningful connections with others?
- Am I able to describe the opposite of loneliness?
- Can I think of one small way that I could create a feeling of connection for myself?

Take the time to sit with the questions above and answer them at your leisure. This is not a race; you didn't get here overnight, and you're not going to change your mindset overnight.

Know that feeling lonely when your kids leave home is not only normal but it's also a good indicator that you have a close and loving relationship with them. So please give yourself time, space, and grace to adjust to this new normal.

CHAPTER 8

All the Time in the World (and Not in a Good Way)

"Time moves slowly but passes quickly."
—Alice Walker

While loneliness is a feeling (which we talked about in the last chapter), having too much time on your hands is often a circumstance that occurs in empty-nest households—one that can produce those feelings of loneliness. Remember the CTFAR exercise from chapter 4? This is a great example of the way the circumstance ("I have too much time on my hands" creates a thought ("This is bad") which creates a feeling (and not a good one).

When we have young children and barely have time to take care of our own bodily functions, multitasking is both a way of life and a necessity. But when the kids head off to college or otherwise leave home, and we are left with endless hours of time to navel-gaze, it can feel as though time's standing still.

The twenty-first-century version of navel-gazing involves spending a copious amount of time on social media—scrolling, clicking, and otherwise consuming the content of other people's lives. Sometimes, we can convince ourselves that using our electronic devices is productive, in our best interests even. And with the advent of Wordle, Byrdle, Boggle, and Dabble, we now also spend time guessing a five-letter word while simultaneously competing with our best friends and family for speed and competency. This digital-age phenomenon is not unlike the sewing circles or book clubs of decades past. The difference is, it's most often accomplished alone, without the benefit of in-person social interaction.

If you find yourself indulging in hours and hours of scrolling or online games such as Candy Crush, Angry Birds, or Mario Cart, it might be a good time to take a pause and consider whether you might be trying to fill your time with dopamine-spiking activities that do little to actually improve your life. I am not saying that a well-timed Candy Crush or Wordle session is a bad thing; I am merely offering the suggestion to consider putting down the device long enough to look for other opportunities to connect with fellow human beings in person.

This was where I found that making a list of home

projects, places I wanted to visit, and things I wanted to do helped me realize that there are so many other ways to fill my days. If you put your mind to it, I bet you can make a list of 100 things you would like to do—a sort of bucket list (minus the need to summit Mount Kilimanjaro or skydive, if you're at all like me).

Many of my clients find this exercise helpful, but it's most effective when broken down into manageable, bite-size pieces. Take your home, for example. Can you name five home projects you've been putting off? My client Rennie told me that she had been avoiding her basement for twenty-five years. She lived in the same house while raising all four of her children, and during that time she amassed a huge collection of school assignments, art projects, and sports equipment. The thought of tackling this overwhelmed her.

"I just avoid it," she told me. "I actually pretend it doesn't exist. If I need a suitcase or something from the basement, I have my husband retrieve it for me." I asked her if she'd be willing to take ten minutes each day to look into just one box at a time. Reluctant at first, she managed to get through twenty-five boxes in two weeks. "I can't believe how much stuff I was saving and how good it feels to get rid of it all," she confessed.

The basement, the garage, the laundry room, and even the kitchen cupboards are areas that likely desperately need your attention after raising kids for so many years. Come up with five home projects and schedule them. Put them on your calendar by scheduling two hours to dive into one of them.

Don't neglect other fun lists to create. You could come up with five places you'd like to visit. These could be local or even international if you're feeling adventurous. Then, move on to five things you'd like to try. Yodeling comes to mind, as does finger-puppet making (just me?), but make your own list.

Lastly, are there people you've been neglecting in your life because you haven't had as much time to see them as you'd like? Make a list of five people you'd like to reconnect with and plan to see each of them. It could be for a walk, a cup of tea, or a lunch date. Perhaps it will require that you drive or fly somewhere, but we rarely regret making an effort to reconnect with old friends or family.

Especially if you aren't working full-time, it can feel like you have nothing but time. That's actually good news! How you fill each day is what ultimately creates your life post-child-raising. So fill it up with things and people that bring you happiness, joy, connection, love, and fun.

Mina had no idea what she wanted to do after her four kids were out of the house. She had been a stay-at-home mom for over twenty-five years. Being a mom was all she'd ever known; it constituted 100 percent of her identity. Mina told me that she was ready to be "more than just a mom" but wasn't sure where to start in the process of reinventing herself.

Over the next few months, Mina mentioned that she continued to receive colorful brochures in the mail advertising various art exhibitions around town. While she wasn't quite sure why, she kept saving them, tucking them away in a desk drawer. One day, over coffee with a friend, Mina noticed a vibrant invitation on the bulletin board offering a watercolor class starting that very evening. Now, Mina was not a painter. She had dabbled a bit here and there with her kids' projects, but she'd never considered herself an artist. And yet, every time she saw something to do with art, it sparked something in her.

That evening, Mina went to the watercolor class. She told me she was quite nervous and made a deal with herself that she only needed to stay for the first ten minutes. If it wasn't a good fit, she could leave. As it turned out, she stayed for the entire week-long course and has been painting ever since.

This is a good example of how valuable it is to pay attention to the seemingly insignificant signals the universe is sending your way. The brochures for the art class were beacons sent to attract Mina's attention, but had she not been in a receptive mode, they would have flown right by her. She wouldn't have given them a moment's notice.

If something—even something seemingly random—strikes you as interesting or fun, consider giving it a shot! Test it out and see how you like it. You never know; it could end up being your new favorite pastime, and it could become an activity through which you meet great new friends.

As you continue to hone your ability to follow the pull of what excites you, you will become more adept at identifying possible projects and activities that might spark your interest (enough to get you off Candy Crush), just like Mina did.

If you're feeling lonely or like you have too much time on your hands, consider one of the following activities, all of which my empty-nest clients have found helpful:

- Volunteer at a school, church, or hospital.
- Enroll in a course at your local college or university.
- Join a club that sounds interesting.
- Try a new exercise class.
- Consider a part-time job.

While these activities might not be things you end up wanting to continue long-term, they can help you identify something new you'd like to engage in for the foreseeable future!

CHAPTER 9

Creating Connection (Outside Social Media)

"I define connection as the energy that exists between people when they feel seen, heard, and valued; when they can give and receive without judgment; and when they derive sustenance and strength from the relationship."
—*Brené Brown*

Thinking back to the days just after Izzy had left for college and I was bumping into walls, dazed, confused, and alone in the house, it occurs to me that those days weren't unlike the newborn months. You know, the days when it felt like the hours were never-ending, yet you were sure you accomplished next to nothing in an entire day?

I was so starved for human connection that I would engage anybody and everybody in conversation.

Sometimes, I'd chat up the grocery clerk at King Soopers. "Nice nose ring!" Other days, I contemplated asking my regular Amazon delivery guy if he would like to come in for a cup of tea.

This may sound ridiculous, especially to those who know me and know that I have a large and generous group of friends. But even still, I felt...lonely. I didn't realize how much of my days and weeks over the past eighteen years had been filled with my daughter's endless activities.

Without the daily routine of school pickup, driving to and from sports practices, and figuring out dinner for three to eight people, I felt at loose ends. I missed the days when she would jump in the car and tell me everything (and I do mean everything). I felt so close to and connected with her, and when she left, I didn't realize she took not only a little piece of my heart but also my purpose.

After a few months of binge-watching Hallmark shows and ordering every personal development book I could get my hands on, I realized that, yes, I missed my daughter. But more importantly, I missed...ME! Somewhere along the way, while pouring all my love, attention, and focus into raising my daughter and loving my husband, I abandoned my relationship with myself. I have found this to be quite common with moms who devote themselves entirely to caring for their families.

Now, I'm not a licensed therapist or relationship

expert, however I'm sure it was obvious to most people that I had become completely enmeshed (the clinical term for being involved in a tangled relationship) with my daughter. I don't regret how super-connected we are, but if I had to do it over again, I would definitely have made more of an effort to maintain my outside interests of writing, tennis, travel, and reading while raising her.

I wasn't sure what the future held, but I wanted to get a little piece of the old me back while figuring out what came next. I knew connection wasn't going to come the way it had in the distant past: wearing midriff-baring dresses, letting random—albeit cute—strangers sip sauvignon blanc out of my stiletto, or chasing down stories for my newspaper. So the question was, what am I going to do to get back that missing sense of connection?

One thing I learned when I was a Brownie (I don't think we had Girl Scouts where I grew up) was that whenever you're feeling lost, in the woods or otherwise, you should sit down, take a deep breath, and pause. So I did…

The next step was to get curious and ask myself some powerful questions. Taking the time to first create a better connection with myself went a long way toward enabling me to create new, meaningful connections with others. Given that I finally had time to create meaningful connections I chose versus connections that were readily available to me by default (such as the moms of my daughter's friends).

Here are some questions that helped me reconnect with myself before identifying ways to allow my new interests to fulfill me and create some amazing new connections.

- What made me happy before I got married and had a family?
- What did I enjoy doing for hours every day?
- Now that I have time, what could I see myself doing if money and people's opinions weren't a factor?
- Is there something that I've always wanted to do, try, or be that I put on a shelf, waiting until I had more time?
- Besides having a family, what has been my biggest dream?

Dear reader, I suggest you look at the questions above, sit with them, and then write out your answers. You might not know the answers to any of all of them just yet, and that's okay. Sometimes, I think it's much easier to know what we don't want than what we do. So if it's easier, start with a list of what you don't want.

Not only did I not want to return to the sorts of connection I enjoyed pre-Izzy, but I also didn't want a full-time job that would prevent me from being able to travel. I value freedom and flexibility. I knew that I did not want to move right away. And I knew that I did not want to be in a constant state of worry about my adult child. But I did want to create more connection in my life.

As a result, I signed up for my first life-coaching certification. What that six-month course did for me was create a sense of community. As strange as it may sound, it provided a new and exciting reason to get up in the morning. I had videos to watch, papers to read, and colleagues to practice coaching with. As it turned out, I did not become a practicing life coach until 2020, but that initial program sparked my desire to learn more about mindset and personal development, and it introduced me to some of my closest and most valued friends.

Are there areas in your life where you'd like to dive deeper and could pursue that desire while getting to know some new people? Have you harbored a secret obsession with knitting? Have you always wanted to learn how to play mah-jongg, or have you been toying with the idea of trying Pickleball? It doesn't matter what your latent desire or newly acquired interest is or how silly it may seem. If it sparks something in you, give it a shot!

Here are some suggestions if you are craving connection:
- Find like-minded people to connect with (clubs, courses, volunteering)
- Be open to opportunities to connect. Say hello, smile at strangers, pay someone a compliment.
- Make it a priority to reconnect with old friends in

order to see if they're still a fit.
- Pay attention to who or what lights you up, and spend more time with those people or doing those activities.

Remember when making new connections it's important to realize that it may take time and feel a bit out of your comfort zone at first.

CHAPTER 10

Where Do I Hang My Mom Hat (and What Do I Wear Instead)?

"Be open to what comes next for you. You may be heading in one direction and then life brings you another that might be a good thing."
—*Natalie Cane*

Not long ago, I received the following direct message on Instagram:

"Help! I look in the mirror and don't even know who I am anymore. For the last 24 years, I have answered to Mom, Mom, Mom! And now, silence. It's so hard to describe. I used to know exactly who I was and what I was supposed to do, and now it's like the whole world has moved on; our kids are in college, my husband goes to work, and I am just left sitting here wondering what just happened! I keep asking myself, Who am I now, and what is my next act supposed to look like? I am so lost."

It was the last part that struck me most strongly: "If I am not a 24/7 mom, then Who am I now?" Six years ago, that was my biggest question! The answer is a bit of a good news/bad news situation.

The bad news is obvious: Your kids are out of the house, and you're feeling lost, maybe a bit lonely, and like you got fired from your dream job. I say "dream job" not because it was always easy or fun, but because it was something that truly gave your life purpose and meaning, and so many of us love being moms.

But here's the good news: you're still a mom; your job description has simply changed. You're no longer Chief Chef and Laundry Do-er; you're more like a sous-chef. I like to think of myself these days as a Chief Consultant. Gone are the days when you are in charge of every detail of your children's lives, and honestly, that's a good thing! When they leave home, it's a sign that you've done your job.

My clients tell me that they still get the "I don't feel well," "I crashed the car," and "How do I make Grandma's red sauce again?" calls, and of course, you want to be available for those big conversations. But when they don't call on the daily, what stories are you telling yourself? Are you making it mean that they don't miss you? That you weren't/aren't a good parent? That you no longer matter? Or are you patting yourself on the back and saying, "Bravo! My kids feel confident and capable and are off adulting. Yay, me!"

When you've had the job (and, as a result, the identity) of mom for two decades or more, you naturally become accustomed to fulfilling that specific role. In my family, I am the organizer, the coordinator, and the soft place to land when things don't go as planned. My hubby takes on the logistics, financial, and academic roles. Also, he kept his day job after Izzy was born, which allowed him to leave at the same time every morning. His day-to-day life didn't change much when she was born, whereas mine did a complete one-eighty!

I made my daughter my purpose (not on purpose), and my identity as her mom was contingent on me being "on duty and available, 24/7." So when I shifted into the Chief Consultant role, it felt like a bit of a demotion, like I had been forced out of my position without any warning. And most of my clients over the past three years have said the same thing.

Julie told me, "I loved being a mom! I never really thought about what was going to happen to me after the kids left, and it feels as though I've lost my identity even though I know I am still their mom." This refrain is so common; I hear it often in my empty-nest community. The question becomes, How can I reframe my outlook when it comes to no longer being a 24-7-365 parent?

One way to shift our mindset from lack and all the

things that we don't like about this new chapter of our lives is to focus on what is working and what we are grateful for now. Nothing dampens a good pity party more quickly and thoroughly than a healthy dose of gratitude. I know it can feel like that word is overused these days, but the notion of focusing on one's blessings will never go out of style.

Some twenty years ago, the famous Buddhist author and speaker Wayne Dyer offered, "What we focus on expands...so if you want more goodness in your life...focus on what's good." Simple, right? Except for the fact that we all have human brains and are programmed to look for the negative. A thousand years ago, this trait kept us safe from predators, but now we have LifeLock, Life Alert, and 911 at our disposal, so we no longer have to be on high alert day and night. Our brains have sadly not yet evolved to the point that they've gotten that message.

I have tested the idea of focusing on something good—even when it seemed like there was no good to be found—numerous times in life, and I must say, there's something to it.

For example, have you ever embarked on a trip and discovered that your flight was delayed? (Is water wet?) Just last week, when my hubby and I were traveling to Vancouver, our flight got delayed. Bummer, right? Well, yes and no. It gave us an opportunity to have a proper breakfast at a sit-down restaurant at the airport and catch up. Also, when I realized I had left my phone in the car, it gave us plenty of time to retrieve it—major bonus! My options were to focus on the delay's annoyance or pivot and focus on the positives. The ability to look for the good—the silver linings, if you will—is not some woo-woo directive or exercise in toxic positivity. It's a muscle that requires practice to strengthen. Think of it as weight training for your mind and soul.

Start with being grateful for waking up, and then challenge yourself to find three things to be grateful for each day. Again, not a new concept, but such a powerful one! I have been doing a version of this practice for more than twenty years (thank you, Oprah), and it has had a profound impact on my life.

While some people have a fixed idea of what they want to do when their kids leave home, remember that I didn't. As I mentioned earlier, shortly after Izzy left for school, my friend Chris mentioned how much fun her friend was having as a life coach. I for sure had never considered becoming a coach of any sort, let alone a life coach. At that moment, I needed my own life coach! However, after Chris forwarded an email from Martha Beck's Life Coaching program, which just happened to be starting a new session of certification later that month. I was intrigued.

The program initially gave me a reason to get up and do something for me, but it ended up giving me a new career I am extremely passionate about.

I had no idea that that program would function as a

lifeline and life preserver. The lifeline is what kept me connected, and the preserver is what kept me above water. It provided structure to my days, accountability to myself and my instructor, and connection with my fellow coaches. This opportunity turned out to be a perfect next step, and the only thing I had to do to find it was stay open to possibilities. You never know where your next opportunity is going to come from, so try to stay open and be curious about how life is working for you, not against you.

While life preservers have a necessary purpose in certain instances and points in our lives, they can also hold us back. Metaphorically speaking, I learned the value of the life preserver (as well as when to hold onto it and let go of it) a few years before Izzy graduated.

I had just finished an hour-long paddle boarding lesson with my instructor, Kevin. I was in my usual uniform: a navy-blue one-piece bathing suit, blue and white wide-brim baseball cap, and my favorite Tommy Bahama flowered sunglasses, complete with a strap so I didn't lose them, of course.

We were hanging out in about six feet of water off Maluaka Beach on the south shore of Maui. I met Kevin and the other staff at The Makena Beach and Golf Club three years prior when I used to go to the beach, but I'd never go into the water. I loved the water, but more as a beautiful painting to ogle and admire than something to immerse myself into.

Kevin and company had patiently watched me go

from barely putting my toe in the water to standing in knee-deep water with either a noodle or a boogie board, all while wearing my bright red, Baywatch-issued life preserver.

I've always loved watching the sun set over the ocean while walking beside it on the beach, and I could even convince myself that a sunset sail was fun—as long as that life jacket was within reach. The thought of being in the water without being able to touch the bottom was inconceivable, as I have an irrational, crippling fear of drowning. Technically, I know how to swim. I took lessons when I was five or six years old. My lessons were unremarkable, and yet I am still out-of-my-mind scared of not being able to touch the bottom when in the ocean.

I knew my fear was grounded in my need for control, fear of the unknown, and a belief that even though I knew how to swim, I might drown. As Kevin and I sat on our boards talking, I suddenly had a wild idea...

"Kevin, what do you think about me taking off my life preserver," I asked half-jokingly.

"Sure, you could do that if you wanted to," he responded.

I thought about it while studying my surroundings. We were bobbing gently on our boards, maybe fifteen yards from the shore. If needed, I could probably touch the bottom with one large breaststroke. I could do this.

I slowly started to unlock the safety snaps across my

chest. It was less of a strip tease scenario and more of a "Here, let me take off my bulletproof vest and jump in front of a firing squad" production. It felt dangerous and wholly irresponsible.

Eventually, I was able to slip my life preserver off, but quickly proceeded to hold it in a death grip to my chest, like Meryl Streep did with her daughter in *Sophie's Choice*.

Every few minutes, I attempted to extend my arms slowly towards Kevin to hand him the life jacket, only to just as quickly snatch it back.

This went on for about five excruciating minutes until Kevin finally said, "It's okay, Allie, you don't have to give it to me; we are fine just floating here." He was sneakily using toddler-level psychology on me, and it worked. I immediately felt the pressure lift. Kevin's easy-going nature and permission to not give him the jacket gave me the space and courage to hand it over, very slowly.

Once I did, I felt elated! I had accomplished the impossible. I was sitting on my paddle board without a life preserver for the first time, and I felt like I was on top of the world.

My bliss was short-lived.

"Now fall off your board," Kevin commanded.

"On purpose?" I asked.

"Yes! There's really no point in giving me the life preserver if you're not going to get in the water," he responded.

I inhaled deeply through my nose and breathed out in big huffing bursts, just as I did when I was giving birth, trying to psych myself up.

You would think I was about to jump off a 300-foot cliff into the abyss, tethered by a thin, fraying bungee cord. But no. I was attached to my paddleboard by a sturdy rubber leash, floating in just six feet of water.

After five more minutes of psyching myself up, I launched myself backward into the water. Splash!

"Kevin!" I screamed as I surfaced.

"Allie!" he echoed.

"I float!" I yelled." I am a floater!"

"Yes," Kevin said patiently, "Allie, you do float."

"You don't understand, I thought I was a sinker," I said. "I thought that without my life preserver, I would go straight to the bottom."

But there I was, happily floating on my back like an otter, my blue-painted toenails poking out of the water. I didn't even have to struggle to keep my entire torso floating.

"Do you want to go back out without your life preserver?" Kevin asked.

"Oh no," I replied. "I need to sit on the beach and process this. You have no idea. I am having a mind-blown moment!" What I realized at that moment was that I had been holding on to a belief that "I am a person who sinks without a life preserver" without any evidence that it was true and having never questioned the belief.

It caused me to wonder about how many other thoughts I accepted as fact, and in how many other ways I had been holding myself back, keeping myself safe and limiting myself from a place of fear. I recognized that I'd come to believe I was too old to be a book author, life coach, and speaker. Also, that I didn't have the knowledge for the capability to figure out how to start and run my own business.

Holding on to both of these beliefs kept me safe, but it also kept me small. The old Allie was trying to protect me and keep me from uncomfortable and challenging situations. But it wasn't until I did my first Zoom call, held my first webinar, had my first TV appearance, or was a guest on numerous podcasts that I realized that my desire to help, to create, to empower, and to inspire was greater than my need to stay safe and small.

This is not to say that everything I tried worked out perfectly. There were many mishaps and missteps along the way. But the more new and different circumstances I survived while learning a lesson or a new strategy, the more I was able to see the value of tossing away the life preserver (in other words, getting out of my comfort zone) as an incredible opportunity to grow, learn, and expand myself and, in turn, help others.

Letting go of my actual life preserver that day in Hawaii was (unknowingly at the time) a big first step in my new life. It taught me to recognize those moments when I was relying on a metaphorical life preserver, one that was holding me back more than keeping me safe. I allowed myself to feel fear and uncertainty about certain situations, but I didn't let it stop me from pursuing my dreams and desires, no matter how big or small.

My question to you, dear reader, is when was the last time you pushed yourself or allowed yourself to be extremely uncomfortable in order to try something new? Further, when was the last time you looked at an old belief, one you've held onto for dear life because it kept you safe but now realize it may not be true and may, in fact, be holding you back from what you really want?

Let's discover who you are today and what's holding you back. I'll toss out a few questions to help jog your creativity. It's okay to take some time to deeply consider your answers.

Are you an extensive reader? A neighborhood walker? A yoga enthusiast? An inventive dinner maker? What else can you come up with? What if I could wave my magic wand, and you could suddenly become anything in the whole world, what would you wish to become?

For some, this exercise is exciting; it opens them up to all kinds of possibilities. For others, however, the choices are either endless and cause overwhelm, or they cause people to feel paralyzed because nothing comes to mind.

I did this exercise with a client named Emily, who

confided in me that she's always wanted to be an actress. "But I am forty-nine years old, so I think that ship has sailed," she lamented. "Not so fast," I replied. She doesn't live in Los Angeles, so being a "Hollywood actress" might be a challenge, but there are many other options available to her. We brainstormed and came up with a few alternatives: regional plays, summer stock, acting lessons, being an extra in movies, and looking into local castings for commercials, movies, and plays.

Emily was ecstatic about the possibilities we came up with. She had assumed that her childhood dream was a bust since she didn't pursue it in her twenties and hadn't really allowed herself to think about it since. "I have been so busy, first with the babies, then the business of the teens, and now that they're all in college, I can finally take a moment to consider what I used to dream about and what I want to do now."

Emily is similar to most women I talk with. She loves being a mom, but once her kids left home, she realized she'd all but forgotten about her dreams and desires from the past. It makes sense—the business of raising kids is a full-time job, and even if you do remember your dreams, they can seem unrealistic and unimportant compared to your kids' needs and desires.

"Selfish" is a word that my empty-nest moms say they feel about pursuing their desires. They tell me, "I don't want to be selfish. How could I possibly train for a marathon, write a book, run for office, go on a yoga retreat in Bali, or [insert your own dream here] when I have kids, a husband, and so many responsibilities?"

Yes, during their younger years, kids and family responsibilities tend to come first. But what if there were an "and." As in, "and...you matter too." And your desires and dreams are equally as important. Remember, it's vital for your kids to see you not only as a responsible parent but also as a whole person who had a life before they arrived and still has ambitions and desires that might not have anything to do with being a parent. You are their first and most important role model. What you do and don't do matters. Trust me, if you are harboring resentments and frustrations, your kids will feel it. Being a parent is immensely rewarding, and wanting more is okay too.

When your kids see you pursuing your dreams, interests, and callings, you're giving them permission to do the same. I watched as my client Katy started her web design business while her kids were still in high school. "My kids knew that I always wanted to be in the web design space and was waiting for the right time. My son recommended me to his lacrosse coach to update the team's site. It was crazy—my business took off after I did the team's website. It was all through referrals and word of mouth, but if I hadn't taken that first leap long before I felt I was ready, I'd probably still be taking another class or waiting for the 'perfect time.'"

Another thing I want to briefly address in this chapter is the fact that while the adjustment to empty-nest life is jarring for most moms, it can be especially jarring for the mom who has only ever wanted to be a mom. She often feels exceptionally lost during this time, because letting go of her child not only creates a change in her identity, but it also feels like a tremendous loss.

If you fall into that category, I encourage you to make sure you are taking the time to process your feelings. Talk with a friend or find a support group. But above all else, know that these feelings are normal, and nothing has gone wrong, even when it feels like nothing is right.

This reminds me of Lauren, who married when she was twenty years old and had six kids in quick succession. Being a wife and a mother was all she'd ever wanted. By the time her sixth child left home to go into the military, she was in her early forties and had never had a job outside the house. Lauren came to me after her sister-in-law recognized that she was struggling.

"I have loved being a mom, and I can't wait to be a grandmother," she told me. "But for now, it's like I'm in this in-between place of not really being needed as a mom because all my kids are grown up but not having grandkids yet. I feel so useless."

I told her that I thought it was wonderful how clear she was about her love of mothering and how excited she was to one day be a grandmother. We also talked about how she could create that feeling of being useful, needed, and purposeful in the interim. We brainstormed ideas for her volunteering at her church, at her school, and at the hospital. She ended up finding a part-time position at MOPs (Mothers of Preschoolers) at her church. "It was so much fun to help these young mothers and to be around little ones again. I didn't realize how much wisdom I could share while feeling joy just being there for young moms in need."

There are many opportunities available for empty-nest moms who feel their purpose is to raise kids—even when their own kids are "grown and flown."

Here are some suggestions:

- Hospitals have amazing volunteer programs.
- Schools have volunteer literacy programs and tutoring opportunities.
- Community gardens offer opportunities to participate in planting and maintaining gardens and educating youngsters about gardening practices.
- Non-profit organizations often focus on the needs of underserved youngsters.
- Some after-school programs provide opportunities to assist with homework or supervising activities or clubs.

I have found that the key to figuring out which hat—or hats—will fit and feel best during your empty-nest years is to be completely open to all life's possibilities. You never know when or from where an opportunity to connect or to serve will come. Staying open, curious, and flexible is the best recipe for satisfaction in this next chapter of life.

Keep your eyes open for ways to connect with other empty-nest moms by considering the suggestions above, but also use this time to get quiet and really tune into what sparks joy in you. Follow the breadcrumbs. The more open you are to the myriad opportunities this next chapter holds, more apt you are to feel purposeful and content.

CHAPTER 11

Communicating With Adult(ish) Kids

"We must remember that one day our children are going to remember our example instead of our advice."
—*Caroline King*

Do you remember when your child was in middle school and would call or text you between periods to say, "Can you bring me my mouthguard? I left it in the back of Dad's car"? And then, when they were in high school, maybe you'd get a call or text saying, "Hey. Heading over to Harry's house after school. Don't expect me for dinner."

You were privy to their every move because that's how it works when they're living under your roof. Once your child moves out, however, the calls and texts suddenly feel (and perhaps are) fewer and farther between. Unless there is a need for immediate cash or a health emergency, you might not hear from them for days. Let's be honest: this is hard! Even if you're one of the "lucky" parents who's greatly looking forward to having your kids fly the coop so you can get on with your new, exciting next chapter, not hearing from your kids after serving as Mission Control for so long is odd, to say the least.

Many moms complain they don't hear from their kids as often as they would like after they leave home. The group that is most distraught about this fact is usually mothers of college freshmen. I was definitely in that group! It is one thing to intellectually know that your child is away, out from under your roof and your control, and entirely another to accept this fact on an emotional level. There seems to be an innate, instinctual desire to know where one's child is and feel like you can protect them—even once they reach adulthood.

Having coached hundreds of moms through the process of learning to connect with their kids differently and in a way that works for everyone, here are my top three suggestions:

1. If possible, have a conversation about expectations around communication and connection before your child leaves home. Ninety-eight percent of my clients didn't have these conversations ahead of time. Now is as good a

time as any.

2. Remember that conversations are, by definition, a two-way street. Yes, you have certain desires and expectations. But remember that your child is now an adult, and you need to take into consideration what works for him or her too.

3. Establish an initial game plan. For example, my friend Susie talks to her son every Sunday evening at 7:00. This works well for her and her family. Her son has younger siblings, and it's important for them to connect with their older brother as well. Just know that, in most cases, you will come up with a game plan and circumstances will change, so it will be to your advantage to be flexible and accommodating.

A few more communication dos and don'ts based not only on personal experience but also the thousands of comments on my social media posts.

APPROACHES THAT WORK

Be Available (and Flexible)

As you both adjust to new communication patterns, you'll want to be available to your child whenever they need to talk through a big or small issue. In fact, you might be surprised by how many "small" issues there end up being! Realize that early on, calls may come when you least expect it, and at times, the timing of those calls may be less than ideal. Remain flexible as

Expect the "I Hate Everything Here" Call

I loved that our daughter's university warned us about this possibility during orientation, because when the call came, it wasn't so alarming! Being able to react calmly with empathy and a certain amount of detachment was useful. Knowing that the call was "right on schedule" made it easier not to overreact and jump in to offer too much advice and assistance.

Ask for What You Need

I dreaded Thursday, Friday, and Saturday nights during Izzy's first month of college. I knew I'd be up all night worrying about her going out and getting home safely. Finally, we came up with a solution. I would go to bed like a normal person, and when Izzy got home at the end of the evening, she would text "home." That way, when I woke up at 2:00 or 3:00AM, I'd check my phone, see that she was okay, and could go back to sleep. Some of my clients get an Emoji text when their kids make it home each night, and others track their kids' locations for the first few months (with their permission, of course).

Let Them Take the Lead

For a while, my client Jill's daughter called her at exactly 8:50 on Monday, Wednesday, and Friday mornings, slightly out of breath from making her way across the campus. It finally dawned on Jill that her daughter was "using her" to talk to so she didn't feel awkward and alone as she walked by herself to class. Since Jill was a stay-at-home mom, this timing worked for her, and she enjoyed the almost daily connection, even if it was brief.

Choose Your Feelings Ahead of Time

Make the conscious choice to choose to be patient, calm, loving, and open. You can do this simply by declaring how you want to behave ahead of time. The trick is having the intention in the first place and having grace for yourself when you slip into feelings you don't want to have, such as impatience, frustration, worry, and fear. You are human, and this is a process where you will choose and choose again.

APPROACHES TO AVOID

Don't Over-Text or Over-Call the First Few Months

Of course, what works best in this area depends on the child. Receiving calls five times a day is too much for one child, while once a week is annoying to another. Make sure that you check in with your child and find a frequency that works for both of you.

Trust me, the need for honest, loving conversations goes both ways. One afternoon during parents' weekend, Izzy sat me down and asked, "Can you please stop calling and texting me 100 times a day? I feel like you don't trust me. I don't want to ignore your calls and texts, but it's too much!" Ouch!

While it stung, I was so glad she told me how she felt. I wanted her to know that I was still there, but I realized that my parenting had become like a giant wet blanket, and I definitely didn't want that. It also gave me permission to say, "Listen, I have never done this before. Please have patience with me. I am learning, and I will try to back off."

The worry is real, and it's normal, and it can be managed through cleaner communication and a commitment to letting go and trusting.

Don't Over-Comment on Their Social Media Posts

I approached this one the wrong way, for sure. I commented with a happy face on a post made by my daughter's high school ex-boyfriend without realizing I'd committed a mortal sin. The older she got, the less she cared about what post (or whose) I commented on. But generally speaking, less is more.

Don't Be Too Rigid About Rules of Communication

Asking your child to call you at 5PM every Sunday may sound like a good plan, but the truth is that college life is unpredictable. Wouldn't you rather your child participate in a spontaneous flag football game, study session, or other fun activity that arises on a Sunday afternoon than refuse those opportunities because they know you're anxiously awaiting their call? Being flexible, not taking a lack of communication personally, and communicating your basic needs around communication will set you up for success.

Don't Take It Personally

This may be hard at first. You used to be the one who did nearly everything for them, and now it feels like you've been fired.

One of my clients, Lisa, told me that when she didn't hear from her daughter for the first few days of college, she felt like it was a slap in the face. "I couldn't believe that after all I'd done for her, she just shut me out," she reported. I told her I completely understood, and we worked to reframe her thoughts. I offered her a thought that maybe because she'd been there so effectively for all those years, her daughter was confident and capable enough not to need to lean on her so much. She liked that a lot more, and it helped her show up the way she wanted to when her daughter did (finally) call.

⁓

When it comes to communicating with our adult children, another challenge that often arises is deciding what the boundaries are around how much you choose to shoulder their need to talk things through (and for how long).

My friend Mimi shared with me that her eldest son used to ask to "go get an ice cream" when he wanted quality time with his mom. "We'd drive around for a couple of hours, and he would tell me all the things. I used to love that opportunity to connect with him. Now that he's an adult, he just stops by and immediately goes into the kitchen to make a pot of coffee. This is the indicator that I'm about to have a three-hour conversation with him, and although I'm here for that, I also have a million things to do!"

The question becomes "How do I transition from being 100% available to wanting to be connected—but in a way that works for both of us?"

If you know the answer to this question, please let me know! Truly, this can be challenging. I absolutely love talking to my daughter; nobody makes me laugh harder! And, she can be a lot, in a million good and challenging ways.

I remember one year when she came home for Christmas break. She was a junior, and I was working in my coaching business full-time. I was coaching, taking classes, writing copy, you name it.

She stopped by my office and asked, "Do you want to go get our nails done?"

I told her I had calls until 5PM.

"How about tomorrow?" she asked.

I was booked until 4:30.

"Friday?"

I was available between 11:00 and 1:30. Probably

not enough time to get our nails done and, let's be honest, grab lunch.

"You know what?" she said. "I liked it better when you didn't work!

When I asked her why, she responded that, back then, I was literally available 24/7. She said she didn't think she liked this "new version" of me. Fortunately, that was three years ago, and since then, Izzy has become my second biggest cheerleader behind my hubby. But we had to have a number of conversations to get to this place. And still, to this day, I have to say, "Oops! Got a call starting in a bit. You've got twenty minutes…go!"

When you have been constantly available for your child during their entire life, there's going to be a period of adjustment for them when you suddenly have other things to think about and do.

More than anything, I encourage you to remember that this is a new season for both you and your child. Everyone reacts differently to new situations. So be patient. You're both experiencing growth and newness, and sometimes, perfecting the lines of communication takes time.

CHAPTER 12

Enter Menopause: Hormone Hell (and Other Rude Double-Whammies)

"You start out happy that you have no hips or boobs. All of a sudden you get them and it feels sloppy. Then just when you start liking them, they start drooping."
—*Cindy Crawford*

The empty-nest chapter of life often coincides with some physical and biological changes that are typically "gifted" to women between the ages of thirty-five and fifty-five. A lesser-talked-about aspect of the empty-nest journey—and one that creates a lot of extra havoc in mom's lives—is menopause and all the other "baggage" that can come along at a rather inopportune time.

As though it's not enough to deal with your child leaving home and figuring out your new identity, hot flashes, weight gain, and mood swings are also part of your new normal.

As we inched closer to Izzy leaving for college, I remember thinking, "So let me get this straight. When I'm in my mid-to-late forties, my boobs are going to start to sag, I'm going to develop a pooch in my belly resembling a full bag of Doritos, and I'm going to feel like ripping off my clothes like a 19-year-old on 'Girls Gone Wild' one minute and bundling up like the Michelin Man the next? And this will be on top of navigating my child's departure after raising her for eighteen years while caring for my aging parents, one of whom has dementia? Please, sign me up!"

Aren't these supposed to be the golden years? Maybe those happen when you're in your seventies. I can't remember. That's another dilemma: women going through this additional life change often feel like they can't remember anything! Once, I was driving my dogs to the park and realized I had forgotten my water bottle, so I left the dogs in the car (with the car still running), parked out front on our busy street so I could run in and grab my water bottle. Just as I saw it on the counter, I realized I hadn't brought the laundry upstairs, so I quickly ran upstairs to put the clean laundry on the side of my bathtub.

For whatever reason, I then thought, "I might as well take a quick shower before I head out for the day."

I was in the middle of my rinse cycle, conditioner streaming down my face, when I realized I'd left the car running with my dogs in it. Honestly, that was pretty normal for a Wednesday. We won't even discuss the number of times I've forgotten to pick up specific groceries or go to doctor appointments, and I definitely have a block in my brain when it comes to going to the dentist, but that may be unrelated.

Back to menopause. While I don't intend to be sexist, you can bet your sweet bippy that if men went through menopause, a cure would have been identified two hundred years ago. As women, we are able to handle so many things and juggle so much and we have such a high tolerance for pain that menopause simply has been accepted as "just another blip on the radar."

But let me tell you, when menopause collides with becoming an empty nester, it's like a nuclear bomb has gone off in our armpits as well as our hearts. We ride the hormonal wave of excitement and glee about the new hobby we've decided to try out of desperation, simply because they are canceling "Gilmore Girls." It's just another Monday, Wednesday, or Friday on the hormonal calendar.

I don't know why I thought that menopause was something that was going to last maybe a year or two, max, but I'm now going on a decade of menopausal symptoms: forgetfulness, hair loss, adult acne, intermittent sadness co-mingled with rage, sleeplessness, and yes, both hot and cold flashes!

While this isn't a book about menopause specifically, the fact is that the collision of this life change with the "kids leaving home" life change is enough to make my hot, sweaty heart melt even faster—especially when I hear from my clients how much they are beating themselves up over not being able to control their moods, weight gain, and brain fog. And yes, there are hundreds of books dedicated to helping us deal with menopause, but I have yet to find one that marries the menopause decade to the identity crisis that arises from suddenly no longer being a full-time mom.

If you, too, are experiencing the unfortunate side effects of all of the above, I encourage you to talk about it. Find a trusted friend, family member, physician, life coach, therapist, book club group, or online chat where you can talk through your experience. Know that you aren't alone. There are millions of women riding this wave right along with you!

Please don't get irritated when I suggest this, but moving your body will help with the side effects of both menopause and the empty-nest transition. Even simply walking around the block for twenty minutes every morning moves the needle in the right direction. Also, absolutely focus on hydration. Think about flushing all the toxins out of your body—those hot flashes can really dehydrate you! Consider limiting or giving up alcohol, caffeine, super spicy foods, and loads of sugar. And, if we're ever together, please don't mention these directives to me. It's very much a case of "do as I say, not as I do."

This chapter only scratches the surface of the additional complexities that can arrive at the same time a child leaves home, such as aging parents and retiring partners. The point is, as you launch your children into their next phase of life, you might naïvely think that your job is done and you'll be walking down Easy Street from here on out. Ha! If my friends and I are any indication of what happens with life post-kid-launching, this couldn't be further from the truth.

I have one friend who has two boys. One is about to graduate college and one is about to get married, and she just found out that she has breast cancer. So yes, maybe most of her parental duties are finished, but now she needs to focus on the real task of caring for herself.

Another friend who has three daughters, all of whom have graduated from college, just had to move her parents into an assisted living facility. She had not spoken with her parents about this, but during the pandemic, it became evident that they could no longer care for themselves.

"It seemed like one day my parents were just fine, and the next day my dad lost his car keys, and my mom couldn't find her purse. It was three weeks before we found it in the oven," she told me. "My husband and I are in our late fifties, and the kids are in their early twenties, so our plan was to take the next five years and travel. That's what we had saved all our money for. But now is no longer the time for travel. We need to focus on making sure my parents are okay."

Those in this stage of life have been referred to as the "Sandwich Generation." As we shift away from taking care of our children full-time, our parents often need our attention. Therefore, we can't focus on our needs, wants, and desires the way we might have expected.

In addition to shifting our focus from our kids to our parents, we're sometimes managing serious health concerns, changing hormones, and the twenty-four-hour news cycle that keeps us constantly on guard.

"It's complicated" aptly summarizes this time of life for many empty-nest moms. There's a lot going on, and I think it's fair to say that few have it all figured out. The best you can do is your best, give yourself (as well as your kids and partners) grace, and have a sense of humor about the absurdity of it all.

CHAPTER 13

Who Am I Married To?

"Remember that creating a successful marriage is like farming; you have to start over again every morning."
—*H. Jackson Brown, Jr.*

"Hey! Do you want to watch *The Thin Red Line* again?"

This seemingly benign question came from my husband of twenty-four years just a few hours after returning home from dropping Izzy off at college. The problem? Twenty years prior, Jim had taken me to see said movie. I was six-and-a-half months pregnant at the time. I don't remember much of it since I only made it through the first fifteen minutes, but I imagine there was a lot of shooting, blood, and gore, because I vividly remember saying, "I don't think this movie is for me. I'm going to step out; I don't feel so good."

By stepping out, I mean that I took a taxi home while Jim stayed and watched the rest of it. It was one of those decisions he may not have regretted in the moment, but after twenty-four years of me bringing it up here and there, he perhaps regrets it now.

And yet, there he was, again asking me if I wanted to watch it! Granted, I was very much not pregnant this time, but I most certainly still didn't love violent, über-gruesome movies. "Does he not know this about me yet?" I wondered.

As it turns out, having a moment wherein we question whether our partner knows us at all is quite common in long-term marriages and partnerships. Preferences, desires, attitudes, and beliefs can change over time, and even though we think that because we're living with someone, they have evolved with us—or at least noticed our preference changes—it's not always beneficial to make this assumption.

Case in point: my friend Meg and her husband have always loved to take bike trips. A few years ago, Meg, who was fifty-five at the time, had a spill on her bike, which left her with a broken collarbone and a sprained wrist. As a result, she announced that she was no longer interested in biking. She traded in her bike shorts for a one-piece Speedo and began taking lessons to learn how to paddleboard and surf.

Lo and behold, what did Meg receive for her sixtieth birthday? Not only a top-of-the-line E-bike but also a two-week bike trip through the Loire Valley in

France. What seemed on the surface to be an extraordinarily thoughtful and generous gift from her husband was, to Meg, a huge slap in the face. She didn't feel seen or heard by him, and it hurt.

"How can he be so clueless? He must be the only person who doesn't realize that I don't bike anymore. That chapter closed four years ago. I feel like I'm living with a stranger!" she told me.

Sometimes compounding the sense that you're living with a stranger is the notion that your spouse doesn't understand and therefore can't relate to what you're going through as a newly empty-nest mom.

Carrie told me her husband, Rick, doesn't have a clue as to what she is going through as a new empty nester. "Rick looks at me like I am crazy because I'm so sad without the kids around anymore. We've always had a decent marriage, but this is just one of those things where his experience of them leaving is so different from mine that I feel totally alone while going through this—even though he's right there."

Even my friend Tina, whom I consider to have a fantastic marriage, has told me that she felt almost jealous and resentful of how easily her husband was coping with the kids leaving home. "It's like nothing has changed for him. Sure, he misses them, but his fundamental day-to-day activities and work have not changed in the least, while mine are completely different."

The feeling of waking up next to a stranger after

twenty-plus years of living together (not to mention experiencing different journeys into the empty-nest chapter) is more common than most of us believe. As mentioned throughout this book, your focus for the past two-plus decades has likely been almost entirely on your kids. Even if you were proactive, had weekly date nights, and connected with your partner numerous times throughout the day, these communications were likely often more about logistics than your hopes and dreams and new discoveries about yourself.

I frequently hear this same experience expressed by clients and friends alike. It's like we all just woke up from a twenty-year dream and have begun to rub our eyes, yawn, stretch, and take a look around. Once fully awake, we wonder whether we recognize where we are (and still like it).

This is not to point out what you've done wrong in your marriage. It is to remind you that at this point, you have an opportunity not only to rediscover why you fell in love with your partner in the first place, but also to reacquaint yourselves with the newer, truer versions of who each of you is today.

Before Izzy left for college, our family had a solid dinner routine. I cooked, Izzy set the table, and Jim cleared the dishes. The night after we returned from dropping off Izzy (before he asked if I wanted to watch the aforementioned movie), Jim and I sat down at our kitchen table as usual. But instead of Jim being on one side, me on the other, and Izzy in the middle, there was what felt like an enormous gap between us. We both just stared at the gap while I tried not to cry.

"Let's scoot closer to each other," Jim suggested. And so we did. But it felt weird. Like a three-legged stool without the third leg. We were going to have to learn to experience life as just the two of us—and be okay with that.

As a new empty nester, feeling like you're struggling to connect with your partner is normal. So first of all, please know that it is not uncommon to feel "off," scared, and uncertain. It's easy to want to jump in to fix the problem or try to make things better immediately. Nobody likes to cozy up with "discomfort and disconnection," but the sooner you allow these feelings, actually allow them and feel them, the sooner they will dissipate.

One of the main reasons people struggle with a feeling of disconnection from their partner is that they never saw it coming. So let's talk about where this feeling comes from and why it's showing up now.

When you spend decades devoted to taking care of your family, you rarely think about "what's next." You're too busy just trying to survive and get through all the things you need to do to keep your kids happy, healthy, and feeling loved.

Why would you concern yourself during that time frame with questions like:

- Are my husband and I still connected and in tune with each other?

- Do I still like him (or her)?
- How will I maintain a connected relationship with my partner once my child leaves home?

I wish I had asked myself these questions and that my hubby and I had sat down to intentionally discuss what life post-kid-raising might look like. We did some chatting, but our conversations were more about my life and identity changing, so it fell to me to figure out how I wanted things to look. Jim was still going to work every day, working out, playing golf, and coming home, as he had been doing since Izzy was born eighteen years prior. The only thing that looked vastly different for him once Izzy left was the way we spent our weekends. In an instant, there were no more lacrosse games, tennis matches, or horse shows to attend.

As a result, we had to figure out whether we still worked without our daughter in the middle, providing the glue to keep us together.

A therapist friend reaffirmed that this kind of transition is extremely common in marriages and stressed the importance of taking the time to "choose again." As a result, during that first year Izzy was away, Jim and I made a conscious effort to get to know each other again.

We decided to take a walk together first thing in the morning (except during winter months) and regularly check in to ensure our schedules allowed for that time together each morning. If our schedules didn't permit our walk at any point, we'd go for a date night or meet for a glass of wine somewhere quiet without many distractions. This small act helped us feel more connected and stay current on the comings and goings in our busy lives.

My friend Nick told me that he and his wife bonded over making dinner. "Now that the kids are out of the house, we can really focus on each other, and mealtime is finally relaxing." He said that his wife sits in the kitchen while he whips up a culinary masterpiece. They enjoy a glass of wine while laughing and talking. "We never had time for this before, and I didn't even realize how much I missed having my wife's attention solely on me!" he shared.

One day, I took a walk with my friend Sarah. She confided, "Andy and I met when we were in college. It feels like we've always been together, and it wasn't until the kids left that I questioned whether this was the best thing for me. I still loved Andy, but I was an entirely different person than I was when we met, and I wasn't sure that we still 'worked.'"

This is so understandable! Twenty-plus years is a long time to be somewhat "estranged" from your partner. Oftentimes, we tell ourselves that we will "get back to being a couple" when we have more time after the kids leave. But even when you've lived with someone for multiple decades, you can't simply assume you're still on the same page about what the future looks like.

My friend Jules was excited to celebrate her fiftieth birthday; she'd been talking about it for years. She wanted a huge party with all of her friends and family a la Oprah's fiftieth birthday bash. Somehow, Steve (her hubby) did not get the memo. "He organized a private fly-fishing lesson for me!" she reported. "I mean, I have nothing against fishing, but who does he think I am, Bear Grylls? I wanted champagne and flowers and to be with all my family and friends. To say I was a little disappointed is an understatement!"

These kinds of stories aren't only shared by empty nesters! Our life partners want to please us, but we have to be extremely clear with ourselves and them about what we want and don't want, especially once we have the opportunity to co-create our next chapter together.

For some, it feels like it's too late to start anew. Sometimes, this can look like a separation or divorce, and that's okay. For others, it's an opportunity to look at their relationship with fresh eyes and "choose again," consciously deciding for a second time that this is the person you want to continue doing life with. It provides an opportunity for a sort of second marriage (but to the same person).

This isn't a relationship book (perhaps the next one will be), but I have learned a number of lessons both from my own experience and from those of my clients. As a result, here are some recommended ways to reconnect with your partner.

Engage in a Getting to Know You (Again) Exercise
State Your Intentions

Start with each of you stating your intentions. For example, perhaps you're looking to reconnect, to get to know the "you" of today, to gain more intimacy, or to see if you're still a good fit.

Ask 5 Questions

Show up curious, as though you're meeting your partner for the first time. Take turns asking each other these questions, or write them down and read your answers aloud to one another. Take your time; there is no bonus for speed.

- Describe me to a complete stranger. What do you love most about me?
- Is there anything you miss from our life before kids? Why?
- If you could describe your ideal day, what would it look like?
- How do you envision the next five or ten years of our lives?
- Do you believe that we can create our ideal lives together? If so, how?

Practice Deep Listening and Suspend Judgment

While your partner is speaking, listen closely (you might learn something new). It's not easy to be open and vulnerable, so make sure you give your partner grace and understanding.

Reflect

Reflect back to your partner something you learned or would like to know more about.

⁓

When Jim and I engaged in this exercise, I learned that he loved our uncomplicated, pre-kid life—the one where we could be spontaneous and choose to go away for the weekend on a whim. I loved that too! I was surprised to learn that he wished we'd followed through on one of our talks about moving to France or Italy for three months. I also learned that my "big heart" is his favorite trait.

Practice Communication

The art of communicating with your partner is possibly the most valuable tool you can cultivate through this entire empty-nest experience. The first order of business is making sure the two of you are both on the same page when it comes to your respective visions for this next chapter. You can accomplish this by engaging in the above-mentioned Getting to Know You (Again) exercise.

Schedule Time Together

Make sure you're making time to be truly present with each other. Schedule a date night or a time to do a fun activity you both enjoy. Besides our early morning walk routine, Jim and I both tried each other's sports: Pickleball and golf. As it turns out, I like giggle-golf with the girls more than I like serious-golf with my husband. As for Pickleball, I'd already fallen in love with the sport and the community, and Jim is a natural (all those years of squash paid off!). It doesn't really matter what you try, as long as you make a conscious effort to spend time together so you can stay current on the goings on in each other's lives.

Plan a Trip Together

Getting out of the same routine will help you have a new perspective on your relationship. This can be as simple as planning a staycation just a few miles away, visiting kids who live out of state, or planning a bucket-list trip. There is something about getting out of your routine and being present in a new environment that can create magical levels of reconnection when we least expect them!

Have Fun in the Kitchen Together

Perhaps you could make a new recipe for dinner or bake a dessert together. Jim and I recently subscribed to Hello Fresh, a meal-prep delivery service, and we have had a blast making our nightly dinners together. For me, it's been such a blessing not to have to decide what we're doing for dinner every night while knowing we'll make the meal together and catch up on our lives simultaneously.

Take Up a New Hobby or Explore a New Interest

From golf or Pickleball to birding or Salsa dancing, the possibilities are unlimited. My friend Brad took up fly-fishing, and to his happy surprise, his bride Mary fully embraced his hobby. Before long, they'd booked fly-fishing trips all over the country.

Take a Relationship Course or Read a Relationship Book Together

This activity can be a bit of a gamble. Most couples who have been together for twenty-plus years believe "you can't teach an old dog new tricks," but you'd be surprised! If a couple is willing and able, they can—even after decades of marriage—still learn a thing or two about each other and about relationship dynamics.

Ask Questions

Every day, ask your partner, "What can I do for you today?" Be willing to ask and receive. Just by offering, you are sending your partner the signal that you are ready and willing to do what you can to ease their load.

Make Play, Fun, and Joy a Priority

Go to a concert, have a picnic, go camping, or grab a mid-day lunch or coffee together. Don't underestimate the power of spontaneity. I am such a planner that I am sometimes guilty of not being spontaneous. But I usually find that when I say "Yes!" to a spontaneous offer, I'm happily surprised by the outcome.

If you're really having difficulties, please consider couples therapy or working with a relationship coach. While it is common not to feel 100 percent connected and in sync with your partner after so many years of looking after the kids, the good news is that you now have the opportunity to shift your focus back to yourself and your mate and discover whether you are still a good fit. And, if you are in sync, it can be a fun and exciting time to create a new life together.

CHAPTER 14

Too Much of a Good Thing(?)

"We cannot selectively numb emotions, when we numb the painful emotions. We also numb the positive emotions."
—*Brené Brown*

Some days still, I wake up and feel…"off," like there's a giant hole in the center of my body, and no matter what I try to fill it with, I never feel satiated, let alone full. There are days when there's simply not enough rosé, truffle fries, or chocolate chip cookies in the world to make me feel better. Do you ever have those days?

Have you ever decided that you wanted to be "healthy" and planned to forgo all sugary treats, alcohol, caffeine, and maybe even your favorite dairy and bread products? In my case, my commitment typically lasts for a couple of days, and then I go on a bender. I don't mean in the traditional sense of knocking back vodka martinis. I'm referring to the kind of bender where you deprive yourself of something and then go off the rails consuming whatever you deemed forbidden a week earlier. During one such bender, I consumed twenty-four mini chocolate chip cookies. In one sitting.

In the coaching world, we call this behavior "buffering." It's when we use something external (shopping, eating, Netflixing) to change how we feel internally. I call it "overing"—over-eating, over-drinking, over-exercising, over-sleeping, over-shopping. The list goes on, but the point is, any of these activities is okay in moderation, but when done to excess, it's often a clue that we're using it as a way to avoid feeling our feelings.

Perhaps this sounds strange. It certainly did to me when I first heard about it. I mean, what would going to Target and buying $600 worth of stuff have to do with my feelings? When I did the research, I discovered that, as human beings, we will do nearly anything in our power to avoid feeling negative feelings. Now, feelings themselves aren't inherently negative or positive, but when we try to avoid a specific feeling (anxious, lonely, sad, bored, or frustrated), we tend to label that feeling as being negative. After all, few of us want to avoid feeling happy, excited, or joyful.

To answer the question: "What does overspending have to do with avoiding feelings I don't want to feel?" I had to dig a little bit deeper. My Target binges provided a high or feeling of satisfaction—but also a false sense of security and control—as I found the perfect throw pillow for my patio. If I could find the perfect throw pillow and feel happy in that moment, why wouldn't I want to prolong that feeling, shop more, and get the perfect gardening set and outdoor mats? Oh! Maybe we need new bath towels. And look, they're having a sale on the new bubbly water machine. I'm sure my family would appreciate that!

Here's the thing: If I were to stop and get quiet—even in Aisle 16 of Target—and simply breathe while taking a moment to assess, "Do I really need any of this? What feelings am I trying to avoid? Is the issue that I'm bored today? Am I procrastinating writing for an hour? Am I frustrated with my friend who didn't do what she said she was going to do?" I would recognize that the feelings of boredom, frustration, or avoidance might be suppressed while I was shopping, but they would still be waiting for me once I'd packed my trunk with overstuffed bags. To boot, I'd probably add shame for overspending to the list of feelings I was having, creating more frustration and annoyance with myself.

Sometimes, we forget that "whatever we resist persists," especially with emotions. A friend of mine, who's also a coach, once reminded me that resisting emotions is like trying to hold a beach ball underwater.

Sure, you can hold it under for a little while, but eventually, that ball is going to pop up and burst out of the water, out of your control. The same is true with emotions. The key is letting whatever you're feeling wash over you like small waves (keeping with the water metaphor). The more you can drop the resistance, the sooner you can move on to feeling how you actually want to feel.

One client confided in me that she was spending her days watching "General Hospital" (I used to sneak-watch it too when my daughter was napping!).

I asked her, "Why is this a problem for you?" Watching TV isn't a problem in and of itself. It's only a problem if watching TV is "masking" or buffering something else. She replied, "I think it's a problem because I want to love my life. I want to be happy like I was when the kids were home."

After we assessed that her compulsive TV-watching began shortly after her boys left for college the previous fall, she admitted, "I really miss my sons, and I don't know what to do with myself all day."

Her overing, when it came to TV watching, was only an issue because she was doing it to cover up the fact that she missed her boys and hadn't taken the time to let herself feel her feelings. Instead, she covered them up with TV-watching.

We know we are overing (or buffering) when the thing that we are doing excessively is standing in the way of what we really want.

Another example is my friend Beth, who wants to travel the world now that all her kids are out of the house. Beth told me that she was excited about her plan to spend six months in Europe, then go on to Africa and possibly Asia. "But," she said, "I have been waiting to do this my whole life. The problem is, I can't afford it anymore."

When we looked at what Beth had spent her money on in the three years since her kids left, she recognized that most of it was unnecessary. "It's like every little gizmo and gadget and makeup product I see on Instagram makes me feel like, if I don't buy it, I'll be missing out," she lamented. "So I buy them. All of them!"

Again, this kind of behavior is more normal than you might think! As I mentioned, we're wired not to want to feel uncomfortable feelings. I won't get into the brain science of it, but trust me when I say that we often default to our primitive brain (the one that wants things to stay safe, easy, and the same) when faced with challenges and discomfort. That's where the overing comes in—the unconscious and excessive shopping, eating, viewing, and the like.

I have my own experience with overing, one that didn't show up in any of the ways I'd seen, so it wasn't easy to recognize until it was too late.

As luck would have it, I hosted my daughter's eighteenth birthday party the same month I hosted her graduation party for friends and family. I also participated in a local fundraiser gala for the arts. All of this happened within a two-week period, which normally wouldn't have been a problem. However, the day after the gala, we embarked on a trip of a lifetime, one that we'd been saving for and planning for eighteen years: an African safari.

My husband and daughter were beyond excited to travel for eighteen hours to frolic with elephants, lions, and hippopotamuses. I, however, was completely spent from a year of "lasts." I was also exhausted and overwhelmed after two weeks of hosting and celebrating. I barely had the energy to pack my suitcase, but on we went. You know the saying, "Same storm, different boat"? Well, that was my experience in Africa. To this day, if you ask my daughter or husband about our 2017 Africa trip, both will tell you it was the best trip ever.

I, on the other hand, felt like I'd consumed gallons of Diet Coke. I was so jittery from exhaustion and anxiety that I felt like I was on the verge of a nervous breakdown. In retrospect, I may have had a few nervous breakdowns during those twenty-one horrific days on safari!

I know, I know, poor me on safari for twenty-one days! But honestly, it's not fun to be on the most fabulous dream vacation if you're stressed, exhausted, and dreading every "once-in-a-lifetime" encounter. I wish with all my heart I could have found relief, course-corrected, or had the sense to cancel, but I didn't, and it ended up nearly killing me.

I won't bore you with the details of all the crazy animal sightings, near-death experiences, or perilous helicopter and five-person plane rides I endured, but I will say that by week three, I was done. When we boarded our flight from Cape Town to Frankfurt, I was not feeling great. I was tired, my stomach hurt, and I desperately needed my own bed.

About an hour into our flight, I began experiencing a violent upheaval from both ends, lasting the entire sixteen-hour flight. (I apologize to my queasy readers for the visual!) I was so dehydrated and dizzy that I was taken from the airplane in a wheelchair to the Frankfurt airport infirmary. I was given bags of saline via an IV, and the airport doctor determined I needed to go to the hospital by ambulance. Since I arrived in Europe extremely sick, having traveled all over Africa, there was concern about my having contracted an infectious disease: Malaria, Zika, or Ebola, to name a few possibilities. Thankfully, this was three years before Covid.

Once I arrived at the hospital, they quickly whisked me into quarantine. The fact that my room did not have a bathroom was unfortunate, however they thankfully provided a wheelchair complete with a bedpan (I kid you not). My husband, who always maintained that most of my maladies were in my head (in the past, he may have been correct), would not adhere to the hospital protocol of wearing protective equipment. Instead, he sat on a small school chair, tipped back against the wall, napping as various doctors and nurses in their white hazmat suits came in and out over the next six hours, drawing blood and taking my temperature.

Fortunately, Jim had the presence of mind to send Izzy directly to our hotel in Frankfurt. The next day, she flew back to Denver by herself. The irony is not lost on me that I had watched, monitored, and controlled every aspect of my daughter's life for the previous eighteen years. Now, here we were, sending her home willy-nilly with no parental supervision; obviously, I was not of sound mind!

After twenty-four hours without finding a discernible African virus in my system, I was allowed to leave the hospital and go to our hotel, where we'd stay for the next week. A day later, Doubting Thomas (I mean Jim) came down with the same virus. I may or may not have felt a bit vindicated.

For the next week, we stayed in our hotel room. Remember, this was 2017, before quarantining was a regular occurrence. We dined on chicken broth, oatmeal, mashed potatoes, and ginger ale. After about a week, Jim announced we had to go home. A quick visit from the hotel doctor confirmed that we were fever-free and able to travel, although it gave me pause when she gave us two pairs of adult diapers for the nine-hour flight home.

I thought all my maladies, problems, and heartache would disappear when I touched US soil. As it turned out, it wasn't that simple. After a few days, my husband bounced back to his old self and could return to working, golfing, and exercising as usual. I, however, continued to have odd symptoms: lethargy, anxiety, and a general malaise about life.

Still, we crossed off every single item on the list for Bed, Bath & Beyond, Target, and Pottery Barn, and before long, my daughter was packed, organized, and ready to go. Me, not so much.

Concerned about my health, my sister flew in from California. After spending a few days with me, she suggested that she would be taking me to a wellness center to rest and recover.

I was shocked when my husband agreed, saying, "You should go and stay as long as you need." My daughter was not as accommodating. If I went, it would be the first time I had put my needs before hers in eighteen years. I would mean missing her last horse show and the last two weeks of summer vacation before she went to college.

Not going didn't seem like an option. I packed a few pairs of sweatpants and a couple of T-shirts, grabbed my favorite-colored pen, hugged my husband and daughter, and went to California to reset my nervous system and rest my weary body. My adventures there are for another book, but suffice it to say that the lessons I learned from taking that time for myself eventually gave me the desire and ability to help others—especially empty-nest moms.

On a happy note, less than two weeks later, I flew to Arizona to move my daughter into her freshman dorm. I had taken some time to reconnect with myself and learned how to put my needs first, or at least on the list somewhere, as I began mapping out my next chapter.

If we are able to take a moment and step back from our overing activities, get quiet, and make space to be able to notice and then feel what's beneath the frenetic activity (it's usually a combination of fear, worry, uncertainty, sadness, anger, frustration, or another not-so-great feeling, we realize that emotions pass, like rainstorms. They may feel enormous in the moment, but if we are willing to sit with them for five or ten minutes, they usually pass. At that point, we no longer need the overing behavior. This, my friend, is so empowering! We realize that we are not at the mercy of our emotions. We can feel hard things, survive, and then move on to what we actually want to feel, create, and do in the world.

TRICKS FOR AVOIDING UNNECESSARY OVERING

Be Self-Aware

Notice when you are out of balance. Are you spending an unusual amount of time sleeping, watching TV, or exercising? Are you eating or drinking to excess? Awareness is the first step.

Assess the Truth

Pause and ask yourself, "What is making me feel uncomfortable? What feelings am I trying to avoid? What circumstance feels uncomfortable or out of control? Am I in denial or avoidance? If so, why?" After you've identified these areas, decide whether you're willing and able to simply feel those uncomfortable feelings rather than engaging in overing to avoid them.

Feel the Feelings

Make space in your day to feel. You can do this early in the morning or late at night. Take a moment and allow yourself five minutes to feel the uncomfortable feelings.

Release the Feelings

Let those feelings go, and trust that things are going to work out as they should. Accept that life is not supposed to feel comfortable, easy, and joyful every single day. Without the contrast of disappointment, sadness, and anger, we might not be able to feel joy, happiness, and gratitude.

In my experience, committing to mindset work and the ability to feel our feelings provides for the most seamless navigation of any challenging life experience.

Taking even five minutes a day to create space to intentionally think and feel will set you up to move through challenging moments more quickly and with far greater ease.

CHAPTER 15

Where are Rachel, Monica, and Phoebe When I Need Them?

"A true friend thinks that you are a good egg even though he knows you are slightly cracked."
—*Bernard Meltzer*

Once you are no longer doing daily rounds of drop-off, pick-up, and other various activities, it's easy to feel like you've suddenly lost a key friend group. And truthfully, this "loss" may fly a bit under the radar for a while.

I was recently having a conversation with my friend Liz, a newly empty-nest (and single) mom, who realized that while her core group of friends was never comprised of her kids' friends' parents, there was certainly a camaraderie that she enjoyed day-in and day-out when her kids were younger. She began to consider that she'd perhaps taken for granted how connected she felt simply being able to chat briefly with other moms at drop-off and pick-up, or go grab a coffee while their kids learned how to color inside the lines (or not). As her kids got older, she stayed connected to parents via social media or text, but as everyone began going their own way, the opportunities to chat began to dry up. She'd even lost touch with the mom of her daughter's best friend (since second grade), with whom she'd once enjoyed impromptu shopping trips and girls' nights out, simply because they didn't have the previously common "We need to get together to talk about such-and-such" messages to relay to one another.

"I wondered," she told me, "if it would seem weird if I texted or called them and said, 'Want to grab coffee…just for the heck of it?' What if we had nothing to talk about beyond our kids' social challenges, college admissions struggles, or simply having a few free hours on our hands?" While these women were never "ride or die" in Liz's life, they were a part of her kids-at-home experience. The swift realization that she no longer had an obvious reason to reach out made her feel oddly disconnected, socially.

In my case, touching base two or three times a week with other moms to ask about lacrosse practice, an upcoming school event, or a weekend sleepover was easy. But without these natural touch points, I started to feel as though I had lost valuable connections.

It's important to remember that the issue isn't so much that we're losing friends as it is that our friendships are shifting. Sometimes, these friendships developed more out of geography, regularly being at the same place at the same time week after week, rather than a shared sense of true connection and friendship. And that's okay. Not all friendships are meant to last a lifetime; the secret is knowing which to keep, which to let go of, and how to make new ones.

When Izzy first left for college, I thought back to the beginning of my daughter's life when I met my new mommy friends at various new-mom-related activities. When I dropped Izzy off for her first day of preschool, I didn't know that the first three moms I met would become my besties for the next eighteen years. I also didn't know that when my daughter left for college, these wonderful girlfriends with whom I'd shared countless mommy-daughter playdates and navigated health scares, divorces, and deaths would naturally fade away. There was no significant upheaval; we were all simply at different places in our lives.

Since I have only one child, my empty-nest journey began much earlier than that of my girlfriends. Most of my daughter's friends were the oldest in their families, so even when they went off to college, their siblings kept the nests of my friends much fuller and busier than mine. My friends couldn't relate to what I was experiencing, and that naturally led to a gap in our mutual mom experience.

I felt quite alone in my "new normal," a feeling that was exacerbated by a sense of purposelessness and a newfound lack of identity. This is not to say that all my friends stopped being great friends. We still saw each other on occasion, but their focus was still on raising their kids, while mine was on figuring out what came next. I felt like I was living in an alternate reality from theirs, and my problems consisted of not being sure what to do next with my life and feeling self-indulgent and silly much of the time.

Kaylee had raised her family in Nashville for the previous thirty years. She not only had a gaggle of great friends but also extended family that had helped her raise her brood of seven. When her husband, Joe, was offered an amazing opportunity to open a new branch of his business in Tulsa, Oklahoma, moving seemed like a no-brainer. The job meant double the income, more growth opportunities, and, as he put it, "a fun adventure!"

Kaylee was on board at first. "I thought, when are we ever going to have another opportunity like this to go out and create something new? I was excited. I thought it would be easy to move to a new town, make new friends, and just start over. Boy, was I wrong!" She had no idea how much she took her community, friendships, and local family for granted. Not that she hadn't appreciated them before, she just didn't realize how much she relied on them for support. Not having that support made life quite hard.

"When we moved to Tulsa, I was so naïve," she recounted. "I thought that I could just step out of my old life into a new one, which would magically include loving friends, close neighbors, and a network of people I would feel instantly close with. This didn't happen." She relayed that her first two years in Tulsa were excruciating. She was not only missing her kids and her full and lively home, but she was also missing all of the friends and family she had left behind. "I felt like such a hypocrite. When my kids said they were nervous about going to a new school, I would say, 'Know who you are, put your best foot forward, be open and smile, and you will attract new friends easily.' Ha!"

She would often go to her neighborhood coffee shop and just stare longingly at the other young moms meeting each other for coffee. "I realized that school had given me a natural way to make friends with other moms, and without it, I felt like I couldn't find my people."

It took about two years for Kaylee to find her groove. She joined a gym that included tennis and Pickleball courts. "I used to play tennis, and I loved it; I just didn't ever have time to play. Now, I had all the time in the world but no one to play with. Joining the gym helped me make new friends and connect with other women who loved the sport and were at similar places in their lives. When I say Pickleball saved me, I don't feel like I'm exaggerating!"

Kaylee is like many women who feel that, for whatever reason—new circumstances, a change in address, or simply different timing—they don't have the friendship network that came so easily when their kids were in school.

It's important to recognize that in this new season of life, the falling away of friendships is normal. The old saying "Friendships are for a lifetime, a season, or a reason" is true. Not every friend you make—even when it leads to a decades-long friendship—is meant to stay in your life forever. Simply accepting this fact makes the process of letting go of some friendships and starting new ones easier.

In my experience, the process of making new friends starts with your attitude. If you can approach this process with openness and curiosity, you will have much more fun and meet more interesting and like-minded people along the way.

TIPS FOR MEETING NEW PEOPLE AND FORMING NEW FRIENDSHIPS

Look for Volunteer Opportunities

Volunteering at your church, gym, kids' schools, or an animal shelter is a great way to give back to your community while meeting people with like-minded values.

Join a Club

Research groups or clubs that align with your particular interests or hobbies. For example, if you enjoy gardening, hiking, or scrapbooking, find a group in your area where you can attend regular meetings or get together to engage in the activity you're all interested in.

Take a Class

Communities often offer free classes in a variety of subjects. Maybe you've always wanted to try your hand at creative writing, watercolor painting, or the art of haiku. Check the community website for your city or county to see what's available.

Attend Events

Research events in your area that spark your interest. Is there an impressionist exhibit at your local museum that sounds interesting? Be willing to ask new acquaintances to go with you to these events. Putting yourself out there can feel scary at first, but once you start exercising this new muscle, it will become stronger, and the process will become much easier.

Embrace the Year of Yes

Vow to make this the Year of Yes. Shonda Rhimes wrote a great book, *The Year of Yes*, the premise being that, for an entire year, when anybody asked her to do something, her answer was yes. This will definitely expand you outside your comfort zone and will undoubtedly help you meet new people along the way.

Be Consistent

Consistency provides a surprising way to meet new people. If you walk your dog at the same time every morning, you will encounter the same people on your daily rounds. Over time, you might feel comfortable striking up a conversation with one of them. This also goes for taking a weekly yoga class or stopping by your local coffee shop at the same time each day. Consistency leads to a routine that can eventually lead to new connections.

Anna recently told me that she follows her intuition about making new friends. "If I feel like there is a real connection when I'm talking to somebody, I will simply ask them if they want to meet for tea or go for a walk sometime. We always assume that everybody else has their friendship buckets completely filled, but that's often not the case."

Just as we tell our kids as they are growing up, the key to making friends is being a good friend yourself. Look for opportunities where you can help, speak up, make a difference, or simply care about another person or cause. Be willing to be vulnerable and put yourself out there in new and different situations.

Sometimes it's helpful to own our feelings of loneliness and isolation and look for others to love and support. Chances are, if you are feeling sad and isolated as an empty-nest mom, there are many other women in your community who feel the same. Perhaps you could even start a local empty-nest group on Facebook or in person. Research shows that when an individual feels seen and heard and realizes that she is not alone in her challenges, she is able to make much quicker progress coming to terms with her particular situation, often making deeper connections with like-minded people along the way.

CHAPTER 16

I've Got 99 Problems (and You're Still 85 of Them)

"You don't have to control your thoughts. You just have to stop letting them control you."
—*Dan Millman*

Most parents worry about their children. In fact, if you weren't told, worry is actually born right after the baby. It's just kind of...invisible. Worry is especially present when young adults are leaving home for the first time. Even if we believe we have spent the past eighteen years teaching our children right from wrong, how to properly take care of themselves, and how to be productive citizens, we still worry. We're parents; it comes with the job.

Just as I've accepted that thoughts aren't facts, I've also discovered that worrying is not only not helpful, it can also rob us of the gifts of the present moment.

I had a client, Jean, who told me that the months before dropping her daughter off at college were fraught with what she referred to as terror and worry. "I would oscillate between 'She's got this; I know she's going to be okay. I've taught her everything I can think of' and 'What if she gets drugged at a frat party? What if she doesn't find her people and doesn't make friends? What if she's homesick and doesn't tell us?' It was an endless list of what ifs."

Listen, it's normal for parents to feel anxious when putting their kids into a completely unfamiliar environment, especially when we've grown used to exerting so much influence and control in their day-to-day lives.

The trick is to allow ourselves to slowly step back so that we can allow our emerging adult children to step up.

It's a simple concept, but it's not easy to execute! The key is to convey and communicate confidence to your child about their ability to thrive in uncertain and unknown conditions. Doing this may even feel inauthentic at first if we are awash in worry and fear. But if we can reframe it by "acting as if," it can begin to feel less disingenuous.

When Izzy left for college, I was absolutely petrified that she was unprepared to take care of herself, and that without my guidance, protection, and daily parenting, she wouldn't survive. I knew on some level that this was ridiculous, but it felt very real at the time. I was also quite aware that conveying these fears to my daughter would undermine her confidence, and I didn't want that. So as much as I could, I borrowed confidence from my sisters-in-law as well as some friends who had gone through this transition years before.

As we moved her in, I was able to keep my anxiety and panic at bay by focusing exclusively on the present moment: "Okay, now we are unpacking boxes," "Now I am organizing the sock drawer," "Now I am making up her bed." I tried to stay present by focusing on what was actually happening instead of what could happen in the future. This worked pretty well for move-in day, and the day's overall chaos helped distract me as well.

It was later that month, when her being gone really settled in, that I had to "manage my mind" more intentionally. My neighbor told me, "When they leave, you have just to let go. You did everything you could; it's out of your hands now, and it can be freeing if you let it be."

Clearly, I wasn't ready to let go entirely. I still wanted daily check-ins. I wanted a play-by-play accounting of the day. "How are your classes? Are you making friends? Eating well? Getting enough sleep?" It was as though my heart didn't believe that it was safe to let go, no matter how many times my brain logically said, "It's time." In order to protect my own well-being, I had to make a few adjustments, such as deleting Snapchat so that I didn't have to witness the 3AM frat party photos. Freshman year was the worst. Everything was new, and much of it seemed scary, harmful, or potentially dangerous. It was a delicate balance of allowing and ignoring while still guiding and supporting.

Fortunately, we all survived the year, and when her sophomore year began, I was better prepared for the lack of uncertainty and loss of control over her day-to-day life. The miracle of slowly letting go of the rope and a daily focus on my daughter's life was that my life became so much more interesting and fun. I had begun coaching, writing, traveling, and connecting with other amazing women. I no longer felt the need to fully control my daughter's life, which was a blessing for both of us!

Worrying often feels both involuntary and productive. As a recovering worry-wort (though my hubby and daughter may disagree about the "recovering" part), I understand that worrying often feels like something we just do, much like breathing. But I will offer that you have a choice: to notice when you are worrying, hit the pause button, and decide whether the worrying is serving you or is simply habit, a default emotion. I challenge you to go beyond worry and reach for empowering emotions such as gratitude, confidence, hope, and love. Although they don't completely wipe out the worry, they can co-exist with it and make a daunting situation that much more manageable.

CHAPTER 17

Yay, You're Home! (How Long Did You Say You're Staying?)

"You see much more of your children after they leave home."
—*Lucille Ball*

Ironically, so many moms say that all they want is to have their kids back at home, under the same roof. But then it happens, and after a week or two, they're wondering how to cope or outright get them to leave! Believe it or not, I have absolutely felt the same way.

Your child may be returning for a weekend, a few weeks over a holiday break, or a longer period of time, such as summer break. Sometimes kids end up moving back home for a few months—or, these days, even longer—after graduating.

When we send our kids off to college, or they move out and get a job, we don't tend to think about the boomerang effect of them coming back home. Of course we want them to visit, and we want to stay connected to them, but a problem can arise when we fantasize about all these returns as though they're Hallmark moments.

One mom told me she had the whole summer planned out. It looked something like this:

Monday nights would include a long walk after dinner. Then there was Taco Tuesday (of course), and Wednesday was Bingo night. They'd have hamburgers on the grill on Thursdays, and Friday nights would be family night with the neighbors. Saturdays were to be filled with hiking, fishing, and picnicking, and on Sundays they'd make an amazing pot roast and play games after dinner. It sounded so fun, but I feared she was setting herself up for disappointment.

Later, she reported that she barely saw her kids at all, given how busy they were reconnecting with their friends. "Basically, they slept here," she said. "I was disappointed that all my plans for us didn't work out but still happy to have them home."

Despite the way we see it in our mind's eye, here's how most kids' returns look in reality:

They breeze in and out like tornadoes, leaving strewn shoes, water bottles, and sweatshirts in their wake. Family plans take a back seat to get-togethers with their friends. Sleep and the consumption of huge amounts of food are their biggest priorities apart from socializing. This isn't to say that there won't be amazing moments scattered throughout, but in talking to my clients and friends (and through my own experience), I'm confident advising you to lower your expectations in order to prevent a good bit of heartache.

Just a reminder: Bonding can be as quick and simple as going to the car wash together or catching a few stolen moments in the line at Starbucks. The key is to be present, open, and flexible. You never know when a moment of connection will arise, and you don't want resentment or hurt feelings to block these great opportunities.

Angie told me she was anxious about her college-age son coming home for the month of December for the holidays. She conveyed that she had kept a very strict household when her kids were growing up. She worried that, while at college, her son was used to having his freedom and independence, and as a result, they may knock heads over the house rules. In addition to encouraging her to have conversations with her son before he arrived home, we also talked about what she could do to minimize her unease.

I encouraged Angie to wake up each day both in advance of her son's arrival and while he was home and decide who she wanted to be and how she wanted to feel that day. She told me she wanted to feel happy, connected, and loving towards her son. She wanted to focus on being grateful for the time she had with him at home, for the person he was becoming, and for his health and well-being. Each morning, Angie would focus on those thoughts, deciding who she wanted to be ahead of time and letting go of her need to control her son's behavior.

In January, Angie reported back that it had been an incredible visit. There were a few bumps in the road, but because she had already done the foundational work of choosing ahead of time how she wanted to show up and how she wanted to think and feel, it was more a matter of getting back in alignment with those choices.

Angie is not a unicorn. Deciding how we want to feel and focusing on that goal is an approach that each and every one of us can incorporate. It is simply a matter of retraining our focus, pausing, and practicing tuning in and listening to our wisdom.

Some suggestions to avoid pitfalls:

Have Realistic Expectations and Be Flexible

Yes, kids will be incredibly happy to be home. Yes, they'll want to see you. But more than that, they'll want to kick back, relax, and see their friends.

Especially with first-year college students who've had a taste of newfound freedom and are under the impression that house rules are something of the past, the willingness to be flexible comes in quite handy. Gone are the days where you get to talk at your children. You may still convey the house rules and expect them to be abided by, but at this juncture, it's important to hear your adult kids' needs and wants as well.

If we've learned anything in the last few years, it's the importance of being flexible. I love a good list and a good plan, and I appreciate it when everything goes off without a hitch. But it's not realistic to expect life to work out that way, especially when a holiday involves multiple other people. So it's a good idea to think ahead of time about what's truly important and what's not, as well as what you're willing to let go.

Communicate and Don't Assume

It's extra important at this time to let your kids know if there is a specific activity or experience that's really important to you. Don't assume that they already know it. For example, the day after Thanksgiving, we get our Christmas tree. This is a tradition for us, and I expect my daughter to be not only physically present but also mentally present—not on her phone texting friends or scrolling social media. This isn't an experience to bring friends to. It's an immediate-family-only activity. I make sure to remind her of this each year before she comes home for the holiday so no one is blindsided by changed plans.

I have 100 examples of ways I did not follow the above tips. I really needed these six years ago! I keep a running log in my mind of ways I messed up. I jokingly refer to it as my "If I'd known better at the time,

I would've done better!" list. I also think it's important to give ourselves grace and move on. So please know that if you're reading this and realizing you've made all the missteps along the way, now is a perfectly good time to change your behavior.

Another shift parents may not anticipate until it's on the schedule is a child bringing home his or her new significant other and not being sure how to navigate it.

When Izzy was nearly finished with her first semester at the University of Arizona, I mentioned to my friend Lou that she would be coming home with her new boyfriend in tow for a few days, and I wasn't sure how to handle what felt like an awkward situation. I had met him briefly when I visited her the month before, but still, this seemed…big!

"Oh my god," she said, "What are you going to do?" Sometimes when I get really stressed, I curse. Or sing, Sometimes both. So I answered her with a sing-song "Oh shit…oh shit…shit, shit. I don't know." I then proceeded to break into song to the tune of the "The Twelve Days of Christmas."

"On the first day of college break my daughter gave to me…"

"Wait! I think I've got something!" I said. I immediately hung up and continued composing.

Within thirty minutes, I'd written the full song.

That's right—I wrote and recorded "The 12 Days of College Break" in less than an hour. The little ditty included the following gifts, bequested by my

daughter:
- 12 friends for beer-pong
- 11 sleepless nights
- 10 kids for sleepovers
- 9 sleeps 'til noon
- 8 missed appointments
- 7,000 selfies
- 6 loads of laundry
- 5 "I'm so bored"
- 4 parking tickets
- 3 family dinners
- 2 bad grades

And the finale…wait for it…"the news of a brand new *he*!"

Writing and recording this song was one thing, but I didn't stop there. When Izzy's girlfriends popped over to meet her new honey, I thought it would be "funny" if we sang it to them as they arrived from the airport.

I must give Izzy and Nick credit. They were great sports about the whole thing. They shook their heads, laughed, and then quickly left to continue their reunion at less awkward homes. Nick, God bless him, is still part of the fam—he knows Izzy comes by her zaniness honestly—and seems to actually find us funny!

In retrospect, I wouldn't wholeheartedly endorse this type of behavior. I got lucky having Nick on the receiving end; I doubt too many other new boyfriends would be so gracious and laugh it off.

The point is, meeting our kids' significant others can be stressful. I would say that having a "less is more" approach is usually a safe bet.

Another dynamic to consider is how your older children coming back affects younger ones who may still be living at home. Consider a time when you went with your spouse to his parents' home. I remember doing this years ago with my hubby to visit his unbelievably sweet parents in Canada. I also remember my husband reverting back to "King James," where he essentially expected his mom to wait on him hand and foot. Being the eldest of six kids, he was used to being doted on. This was not the man I married, the one who carried out household chores like a boss and was always helpful and gracious.

This is what it often looks like when older kids come home. There is an unconscious backsliding into old pecking orders and patterns. Younger kids who may have felt more "grown-up" and empowered since the departure of their older siblings are quickly put in their place. It can feel a little wonky and chaotic while everyone figures out where they fit in.

Lucy told me that she felt like her quiet, serene home turned into a war zone when her kids came home for a short break. "When Jack and his brother came back for the holidays, we were so excited. Everything was fine for about three days, and then the squabbles began," she said. "I know they love each other, but they quickly get on each other's nerves, and then Brad and

I get upset because we just want everyone to get along and enjoy our short time together."

It's normal for the dynamic of the household to change as kids come and go. The trick is to keep your expectations at bay and make sure that you are spreading your attention equally between younger and older kids.

Our adult kids can also return home unexpectedly, and as much as we welcome them in our hearts, these returns can also upset the apple cart, so to speak. "We thought our daughter had a great first semester her freshman year, but when she was home for the holidays, she confided in us that she was depressed and really didn't want to go back after the break," a client told me. "We were conflicted as to whether we should push her to go back and see it through or let her stay home."

As it turned out, they let their daughter stay home and found her a great therapist, but it wasn't without much soul-searching on their part. "We wanted to do the right thing. We didn't want to enable her, but we were also very mindful of how difficult it has been for kids these last few years."

Adult kids living with their parents is more common than you might think. According to a 2022 Prudential Financial poll, approximately fifty-eight percent of US young adults live at home. As much as many of my empty-nest moms think this would be a huge blessing, it still impacts all areas of parents' lives:

financial, social, and emotional.

The best way to face this new reality is to set up clear expectations and boundaries. This is where communication is key. Remember that these kids are used to having freedom, so try not to micromanage their comings and goings. It's also important that, as members of the family, they contribute to the household via chores and responsibilities.

There's no reason to freak out when your young-adult child moves back home for a bit, should that happen. They may just need a moment to reset. It is highly unlikely that they will be with you forever. Setting up a timeframe for how long you are willing to support your child is wise. If you convey this information upfront, you mitigate misunderstanding and resentment that might creep in from unmet expectations.

One last thing: It's okay to love having your kids home and be happy to see them return to their homes and lives. I assume it's like watching the grandbabies—so grateful and happy for the time together, but a relief to give them back to their parents. Both can be true at the same time!

CHAPTER 18

All the Single Ladies: Put Your Hands Up!

"I think moms, single or not, put a lot of pressure on ourselves trying to balance it all. It's *never* going to be perfectly balanced—the sooner you know this, the sooner you can relieve some of the pressure you put on yourself."
—*Denise Richards*

This chapter is for my single mamas. As you know by now, I'm not a single mama, so I don't have personal knowledge of the highs and lows of parenting a child as a single mom or experiencing the empty nest as a single mom. However, I have spoken to many women who are single, and I've had numerous clients who've shared their experiences with me. This chapter is based on those conversations.

Whether we're talking about being married or being

single, the phrase "the grass is always greener" seems to apply. Many of my single girlfriends tell me that once their kids have all left home, they want a partner to ease the burden of day-to-day life and quell the loneliness that they feel in the evenings and on weekends. By the same token, many of my married friends and clients share that their ideal life is one in which they have sole control of their home environment: their kitchens, TVs, bedrooms, and bathrooms, not to mention what and when they eat, and how they spend their free time.

It's important to note that there are pros and cons for both circumstances. The key is to make peace with whatever circumstance you're in and try to find the beauty in what's working versus focusing on what isn't working or on what you don't have.

We covered the topic of loneliness in chapter 4, but if you're feeling lonely as a single mom, it can create an extra layer of melancholy. Whereas a night alone can feel peaceful and restorative to an empty-nest mom with a partner, the booming quiet can feel almost suffocating to a single empty-nest mom craving connection and company.

"I used to hate going home after work," my friend Denise told me. "It felt like I was entering a tomb when I walked in the door. The quiet was deafening and only made me miss my kids that much more!"

Home, which used to be one's sanctuary—the hub of all activity, the place where everyone gathered, laughed, and maybe even cried together as a family—somehow turns into a source of pain as it constantly brings up memories of the past.

Just as every child is different, so is every single mom's empty-nest experience. My friend Molly loves her newfound freedom and has embraced this next chapter with excitement and optimism. "When my last son left for college, I was ready to see what life had in store for me. I didn't know exactly what I wanted to do, but I knew it would include travel, personal development, and helping other women." It took Molly a few years to hit her stride, but she now travels all over the country consulting with hospitals on how best to support young moms. "I combined my nursing experience from twenty years ago with my desire to help moms and literally created a new job for myself. I love it!"

I was thrilled when I heard this. Molly was able to take a skill set and experience she hadn't practiced in over twenty years and parlay it into an opportunity that fit her current lifestyle and her dream life. But of course, being able to turn lemons into lemonade in this way isn't always possible.

I heard from my client Alma that she felt the cumulative effect of no longer having her kids home, a decades-long experience that gave her a sense of companionship and support but also contributed to her lack of identity and place in her community. "When you have five kids, you're sort of known in the community as 'The Miller Clan.' As each of my children left, I could feel my identity slipping away. If I wasn't so-and-so's mom, then who was I? Maybe it was my imagination, but I felt like people treated me differently. Like without the kids, I was a nobody. It definitely contributed to my feeling purposeless and isolated."

While Alma is a single mom, it seems that the feeling of "Who am I if I'm not a mom?" isn't limited to single, empty-nest mamas. I have heard the same sentiments echoed by married clients and friends. The difference seems to be that, for some, the feeling of loneliness is sometimes mitigated or dampened by having a partner.

Another friend, Elizabeth, said, "It was very odd to go from coordinating the chaos of five kids to, over the course of three years (two of them are twins), suddenly not be doing it anymore. It doesn't look the way I thought it was going to look, and to be honest, I don't even know how I thought it was going to look. I just thought, 'It will be fun. I will finally have time to do all the things that I've wanted to do.' But that's not how it actually played out."

Amen, sister! This seems to be the common denominator (whether a mom is a single empty nester or married): Our lives don't look the way we thought they would look after kids leave. Even if we didn't know exactly what that picture entailed, we know this wasn't it.

While the experience of single empty nesters is

unique, the truth is that the experience of every empty nester is unique! Whether single or partnered, most empty nesters are attempting to gain footing in this new reality. Your life is yours alone to manage, and that freedom and flexibility can feel so exhilarating!

Should you be a single empty nester, I want to leave you with a list of incredible benefits that come with your status (compiled by my single comrades) that you may not have considered:

You Don't Have to Ask for Permission for…Anything!

Imagine, if you want to buy a new couch, you find one you're in love with and buy it! Want to have ice cream for dinner? No one's expecting anything more substantial. Watch a movie about Italy and decide you want to go? Book that flight on a date that works for you!

You Have the Freedom and Flexibility to do the Things You Want to Do

Sleep until 10AM on Saturday: check! Meet a friend for an impromptu brunch on Sunday: check! Go to NYC on the weekend because you want to: check!

The Grocery Bill is Lower

I'm not suggesting you didn't happily buy $300 worth of groceries every week when your kids were home, but what a shock when your weekly bill goes from $300 to $150. More money for your Amazon necessities!

You Have the Opportunity to Meet New People

It's always a little tricky to be dating when your kids still live with you. Not to mention determining when is the exact right time to introduce them to your new partner? Is it after six weeks or six months? Now that you have the time and the space to date and meet new people, you no longer have to juggle those vying for your attention.

Your Space is Always Exactly How You Left It

When you leave for work, you don't have to worry about coming home to a disaster in the living room and no food left in the fridge. It's one less thing you have to manage; what a relief!

∽

My friend Bridget is a single mom of twins, and she worried about how it would feel to suddenly have the people she cared most about off doing their own thing (and not returning every night, at least for food!). Of course, she missed them when they left for college, but she was also able to enjoy some of the "unexpected benefits" of sharing the house with only her dog.

"I was encouraged by someone I deeply respect to

think about the things I appreciated about being home alone instead of feeling sad about how quiet the house was," she said. "For one thing, there were no more late-night loud video games. I do not miss those! For another, there were no more empty cereal boxes in the pantry or bags of bread with just the heel in them in the refrigerator. They were little things, perhaps, but they helped me focus on the positive aspects of the transition."

I have heard many of my single friends and clients lament, "If I were married, life would be so much easier," or "if I were on my own, life would be simpler." Honestly, I don't know if in your particular situation this is true, but I do know that your circumstances alone don't determine your happiness. It also comes down to how you choose to perceive your circumstances and whether you are open to creating new opportunities within your circumstances. So if you're a single mama getting ready to navigate the empty nest (or already in the throes of it), consider the possibility that what's coming has the potential to be as magical as you decide you want it to be.

CHAPTER 19

So…Now What (Again)?

> "Twenty years from now you will be more disappointed by the things you didn't do than by the ones you did do. So throw off the bowlines. Sail away from the safe harbor. Catch the trade winds in your sails. Explore. Dream. Discover."
> —*Mark Twain*

The empty-nest phase of life can be summed up in one word: bittersweet. As children head off into the world to learn, grow, and create amazing lives for themselves, we, as empty nesters, have an opportunity to learn, grow, expand, and, most importantly, create a fulfilling and purposeful next chapter in our lives.

As you have read, each person's empty-nest journey is unique. There is no one-size-fits-all prescription or even preparation for this time of transition.

My hope is that, more than anything else, you feel more reassured that you are not alone. According to the 2020 census, there are approximately 22.5 million empty nesters in the US. That's a lot of parents who are navigating some form of creating a new next chapter.

Feeling comforted that you are not alone is just the first step. The next is actively choosing how you want this next chapter of your life to look. I hope this book has served as a primer, an inspiration, or a beacon of hope that leaves you confident in your absolute ability to be happy and fulfilled after the kids leave. I promise, you can. If someone had told me six years ago that I would, at this point in my life, be the happiest I've ever been, I would never have believed it!

But by taking the time to feel my feelings, engage in mindset work, take micro but consistent action, and stay open to possibilities, I created my most favorite chapter of life while still feeling connected to my daughter and husband. The bonus was that through my willingness to be vulnerable and my desire to connect and make a difference, I discovered my next purpose: helping other empty-nest moms.

It is my absolute honor to be on this path with you. I'm with you every step of the way!

ACKNOWLEDGMENTS

If I were to list everyone who's ever supported me in my book writing endeavor, it would create a whole other book.

To begin with, "thank you" seems inadequate to express my gratitude to Elizabeth Lyons, my editor, who helped me shepherd this book from sticky notes to completion. You are brilliant, supportive, and hilarious, and now a trusted friend.

To my sweet Ashton, who took me from 200 to 20K+ followers on Instagram in two years.

To Jen Liddy, who saw my potential before I did, wrote down everything I said, and then reminded me I said it!

To Shannon Clendenning, for all things tech-related. Whew! You are an angel!

To Catie Borland, who helped me reconnect to my essential self in business and in life.

To Aimee Gianni, for being an example of strength and beauty as a successful coach and therapist.

For my fabulous coaching peers, Crystal, Jennie, Joanne, Heidi, Jewel, Pamela, Kristine, Christine, Andrea, Jewel, Janet, Brooke, Lor, Patti, Loralei, Cathy, and so many more, whose love and support (and prayers) I've been the beneficiary of for the last three years, and who made my life so much richer! I am so lucky to have met all of you and to have you in my life!

To my writing mentors, Natalie Goldberg, Martha Beck, Betsy Rapoport, and Linda Sivertsen.

To my best girlfriends, Marni, Mary, Melanie, Tammy, Tonya, Isabelle, Izabel, Kate, Kim, Pam, Ashley, and Sindy: thank you for sticking with me even when I was MIA working on this book. I love each and every one of you. I am now available! Girls trip?!

To my beautiful Maui ohana, Mahalo Nui! Again, there are too many of you to name individually, but please know that you all contributed in a big way to smoothing my empty-nest journey, finding my purpose, and expanding my belief in myself.

To my amazing and supportive Canadian family: I think there are now about thirty-two of you, so I won't name you individually, but please know that as a collective I love all of you, especially my incredible sisters (sisters-in-law) Cathy, Peggy, Judy, Elizabeth, and Mary! You are my role models and my family!

To my mom, dad, and sister: thank you for your love and support. And to my remarkable cousins, Catherine and Anne, I love and appreciate our bond.

Is it weird to thank my daughter's friends? I don't care! I love them like my own, and their support has meant the world to me. To Nick, Betts, Kyla, Emily, Riley, Sara, and Natalie. Sleepover soon?! (I'll let you keep your phones!)

A huge thank you to my empty-nest community. To my beautiful clients, thank you for sharing your lives with me. This book is the result of your willingness to share and be coached as well as to allow others to learn from your unique journeys.

A huge shout out to my incredible Instagram following (@AllieHillCoaching)! You helped me believe that I had something important to say and that I could help other empty-nest moms. I love you...and please know, you've got this!

To my small but mighty family, Jim and Isabella. Without the two of you I'd just be a girl in the world. You have given me unconditional love, support, and most of all, purpose. I hit the jackpot with you two. Thank you for being my people.

I'd like to extend a heartfelt thank you to all the people who have made my life easier so I could focus on my writing: Molly, Dorothy, MaryBeth, Angelica, Cris, Robert, Nader, Suzi, and Hector. And last but never least, Peri, who makes everyone's lives better!

Also, a big hug and huge dose of gratitude to my brilliant and compassionate therapist friends: Randi, Kathleen, and Candice, who reminded me that *being* is more important than *doing*, and that empty-nesting can actually be a ton of fun!

And lastly to you, dear reader, this has been such a labor of love for me. It's my gift to you, and it is my wish that you read it, highlight it, earmark it, use it as a guidebook and then pass it on. I can't wait for your feedback, as I'm already hard at work on book #2.

XO,
Allie

ABOUT THE AUTHOR

Allie Hill is a writer, speaker, and certified life coach who helps empty-nest moms feel empowered to find new meaning and fulfillment in life.

Allie's experience as an empty-nest mom and coach enables her to provide a safe space for her clients to create, dream, and discover who they are and who they want to become.

Her fifteen years' experience as a journalist helped Allie become a more powerful coach, bringing curiosity in and using her deep listening skills to transform people's lives. In addition, Allie is trained as a Desire Map facilitator, helping people design a life that aligns with their true values and goals.

Allie has been featured on national television, is regularly interviewed on a variety of podcasts, and shares her knowledge in workshops and trainings throughout the country.

www.AllieHillCoaching.com

Made in the USA
Middletown, DE
16 May 2025

75649075R00116